A Way of Life and Medicine

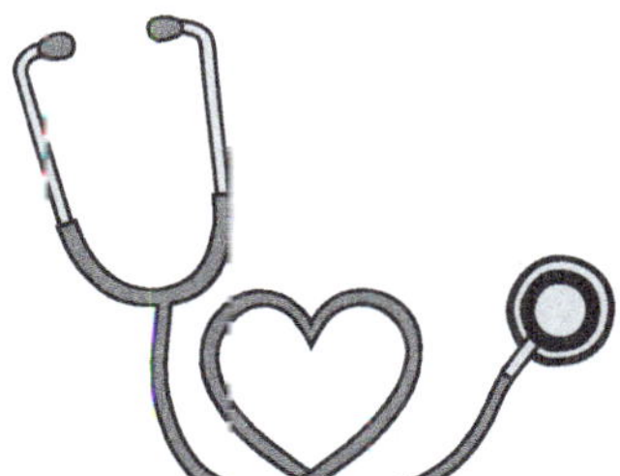

Dr Clive Barker

First Published in March 1997
by
Limited Edition Press
No 2 at 164 Whalley Road
Whalley Range
Manchester
M16 8AW

Second Edition published in February 2020
by
Open Circle Books

A CIP catalogue record for this title is available from the British Library.

ISBN 978-1-909607-20-0

CONTENTS

DEDICATION

This book is dedicated to those who appear herein

ACKNOWLEDGEMENTS

Carole, for giving me time in the evenings to complete this, even when all the kids weren't in bed.

Gillian Hudson, one of my long-suffering secretaries, for typing this work and, with Don Ross's help, figuring out how to use the computer.

Clive Barker, the famous author, for having the same name. Perhaps people might confuse us, and start reading this book thinking it might actually be interesting.

The British Medical Association News Review Journal, for awarding me the dictaphone on which this work was first recorded, for one of my lamenting letters regarding the GP contract.

The Medical Protection Society, the General Practitioner Writers' Association (now the Society of Medical Writers), and Wilfred Hopkins of the Limited Edition Press, for inspiring me to commence this work.

PREFACE TO THE SECOND EDITION

Twenty-two years have flown by since the first edition of this book was published. Where they went is described in my second book, *A Way of Medicine and Life*. That book, and the three evenings at Chorley Little Theatre talking about life and medicine led to some people kindly enquiring about this first book. There were no copies left, and since its second print in 2008 technology has moved on so much it seemed appropriate to publish a fresh, second edition, facilitated by my friends at Chorley Writers Circle.

Very little has been changed from the first edition, which is how I felt when I wrote it at the age of 37. Some of it may seem outdated now, less mature, possibly embarrassing, and the writing unskilled, but it was me at the time, (not that I've matured much).

Reading through this book in preparation for the second edition, I think I learned more from writing it than I realised at the time, and one reviewer called it cathartic.

I am even more aware now how lucky I am to have experienced the life I have so far, with family, friends, colleagues and patients. It is a huge privilege to have tried to look after people who mostly seem to know that I did my best to care for them, and who know that I, like everyone else, am not perfect, and only human.

PREFACE TO THE FIRST EDITION

Why, at the age of 37, write a book about experiences in life so far? I should be living for the present and the future, and not the past. Like some of my patients, hopefully there will be time to look back and reflect in years to come when, possibly, I am less able to do as much at that time. Well, I feel I am living life to the full now and planning for the future, but there are a number of reasons for putting pen to paper, voice to audio-tape, or finger to keyboard.

Like many things in my life my parents spurred me on. Their current research into our family history has highlighted how transient life is. Each one of us gets a moment to shine, and then it's gone forever. In a hundred years I'll be a fading memory and so will most of us be. So, as well as making the most of it while I am around, I would like to leave a little something about our fragment of life, the universe and everything, as we see it now.

In recent years I have had cause to think a little about what life means. I haven't found the answers, only more questions and some of them are here. I am not conceited enough to think that this account will be of interest to anyone other than me, but it has clarified for me some of the reasons I chose medicine, and some of the other paths in my life. If it is of interest to anyone with similar choices to make, or any interest generally, so much the better.

Many people are featured in this book and some of my friends, hopefully not soon-to-be ex-friends, tell me they have their lawyers alerted, but I have not given, and would never give, any confidences away about anyone.

During the development of this work I have been aware of my limitation in the use of English, but it is not supposed to be a work of literary genius! It is just my way of telling a story. We all have a tale to tell and this, with the people I have known, is mine. Writing this book is no big deal. I don't get much time to read myself, but I thought this year (1996) instead of reading a book, I'd write one. On writing the final draft, I occasionally referred to those well-known tomes *The Oxford Mini Dictionary* and *Collins Reference Thesaurus*, though I almost mistook *The 1994 Good Pub Guide* for the latter, which may have been as good.

This work I nearly called *An Ordinary Life*, as just because most of us haven't achieved anything famous, does not mean we haven't done anything with our lives.

FOREWORD

The little boy looked up at me with trusting eyes. Earlier that day I had seen his father, who I thought had a brief self-limiting illness which would shortly resolve. Having explained this, I said I would telephone in the evening to see how he was. I never got the chance. One hour after I had seen him he was dead.

Although that tragedy was to affect many people, it was to affect me in ways I could never have imagined that day. In the months and years that followed I thought much about what one can and cannot do in medicine, and in life, and in death. This book is the result. Everything in it is true.

CHAPTER ONE

Considering I wanted to be an astronaut or a rock star, medicine is perhaps an unlikely eventual choice. However, having a fear of heights and no musical ability (unimportant, I hear you say?) set me back somewhat.

When I was born in 1959, man, and woman, had yet to venture into space. Rock and roll had been around a few years, but from what I have read, post-war austerity was only just ending. Though great strides had been made in medicine, it was only that year that oral penicillin became available, and still two years before the oral contraceptive was marketed. It was before the Cuban Missile Crisis, before John F. Kennedy's assassination and before the Berlin Wall was built. Fortunately, I was too young to know anything about those events at the time.

My earliest known medical ancestor was a Dr Richard Lucroft, a surgeon who lived in Devon until his death in 1742. His son, John Lucroft, practised in St Kitts in the West Indies, where he was buried in 1758. A descendant of John's, Dr Henry Whitworth, who lived from 1817 to 1883, was born in St Bartholomew in the West Indies, and from 1839 lived in St Agnes in Cornwall. We understand one of his sons, William, became a doctor and practised in St Agnes, and another of his medical sons, Edward, was dispatched from St Agnes to Thornborough in Queensland, Australia, possibly because he drank. This is a recurring theme in my ancestry! One generation appeared to be upstanding teetotallers, and the next, possibly disinterested in their parents' staid ways, seemed to have a fondness for alcohol. This in turn puts the next generation off, who may have become Methodists or similar.

My great-great-grandmother was a sister of Dr Edward and Dr William Whitworth and married Cornelius Rimmington in the mid nineteenth century in Selby, Yorkshire. From then until the present day I have no direct medical predecessors, though my father's mother, Doris Rimmington, was, on qualifying at the age of 21, the youngest pharmacist in the country at that time. She had been encouraged by her father who had the chemist's shop in Shipley, Yorkshire. She married my grandfather in 1928 and, after marriage, never worked again. Even though they were short of money and she had nothing to do, it would appear that for her to work was not the done thing! Her husband, Jack, was an industrial chemist. Like many others at that time, he was unemployed after qualifying, but finished up working for Clayton Aniline in Manchester, eventually becoming joint managing director. Jack and Doris had four surviving children: my dad, Michael, and three younger sisters, Lesley, Gill, and Anne.

My grandfather on my mother's side went into the family firm, processing cotton cloth. He and his wife, my granny, had two children: Malcolm, who also went into the family firm, and my mum, Pauline.

My father trained as a dentist at Manchester University, then undertook six months as a house surgeon, earning £8 a week. National Service was deferred for him while he gained this experience. One week was spent with medics learning what to do when he had been hit by a nuclear bomb! We think this was at Weeton in Lancashire, and most of the time was spent playing snooker, which was probably all one could do at the time when a nuclear bomb was about to land on you. In the RAF, he was posted to Jordan, and after the Suez conflict was over, was posted to Cyprus.

My dad is not quite sure where he first met my mum, but it was probably when he saw her in an amateur dramatics production. They both attended each other's 21st birthday parties, and appear to have got things together shortly after that. They were married on 11 April 1957, and then flew back to Cyprus. They appear to have had an eight-month honeymoon, during which Dad worked till the early afternoon, and they spent the rest of the day together. I am glad they got this opportunity to spend time together in what seems, from an observer's point of view, to be fairly idyllic surroundings, though no doubt in reality it had its problems, besides the cockroaches.

On returning to England, Dad joined a small dental practice in his home village of Bramhall, and shortly after assumed responsibility for the practice. I arrived in March 1959, followed by my brother Alec, on New Year's Day 1961. Initially, we lived in a moderately sized detached house in Cheadle Hulme nearby, but then moved to the same house as the dental surgery, where we lived from when I was four until I was thirteen years old. This was a fairly large house in its own gardens.

In the mornings my dad would walk from the dining room through two single doors, one of which was soundproofed with lead, some of which is probably still in my bloodstream, to a world of sterile smells and high-pitched screeching drills, and women in starched white uniforms. Perhaps this fascination with clean smells and uniforms later led to my interest in the medical and nursing world.

Living next to the shop, so to speak, had its obvious drawbacks. Our home telephone number was the same as the practice's, which meant that my father could be called in at any time of the day or night, Christmas Day included. In fact, this did not happen often, and most people's expectations of availability were not as high as they are now.

Some fathers would have careers that opened doors to travel, restaurants, free gifts and samples, or tickets to football matches. We occasionally had free toothpaste or, if very fortunate, toothbrushes. We did, however, get to play on newfangled electrically operated dental chairs. I think my father had ulterior motives, as this special treat was probably organised so that we would get used to sitting in these chairs when he found a new treatment he wanted to try out on my brothers and me. The treatments I particularly remember are a clear plastic fissure sealant, which was painted on to our teeth then set with an ultraviolet light. I also remember a particularly unpleasant tasting fluoride gel application that was applied to our lower teeth while suction was applied to produce a sound not dissimilar to the aspirators inserted during major surgery to clear yards of intestine.

Sadly, all these measures did not prevent my teeth from decaying, and I now have large chunks of metal in my mouth, which I show to my children in the hope that they will look after their teeth better than I did. Admittedly, matters were not helped in the 1960s or 70s by the lack of fluoride in the toothpaste, and by my sometimes clandestine ingestion of sweets, Cola, and hot Ribena.

Dad worked five and a half days a week, fifty weeks a year, bringing his paperwork home, through the leaded doors, for the other day and a half a week. This did pay for a reasonably comfortable way of life for us, and though at times my mum must have wearied of his long hours, she rarely, if ever, showed it to us. My mum's life was, and still is, devoted to looking after Dad and, in those days, Alec and me, and then Guy, my youngest brother born in 1964. Guy was born at home attended by our GP and midwife. Dad popped upstairs between patients to see what progress was being made.

This was the norm at the time, the father not being expected or being cajoled to be there. In the 1990s, of course, the father, if one is identified, is made to feel like a selfish wimp if he is not at least at the soon-to-be mother's side during the delivery. Many a strong man has slipped quietly under the delivery couch during their child's appearance into the world – but more of that later.

Although we no doubt fought fiercely at times, my brothers and I were great companions in those early years. Subsequently, I learned from Alec that his memories of his youth at home are of playing outside with Guy, while I studied in my room upstairs. I had rather rosier recollections, but obviously these are subjective.

We holidayed in a small rented flat in Rhosneigr, Anglesey, where we fed an electricity meter with silver coins to heat us. We played in the sand dunes and the sea, occasionally nearly drowning in a large fibreglass twin-seater canoe in which four of us would try to paddle.

The family vehicle that used to take us on these trips was a succession of Dormobile vans. These ranged as the years went by from 'extremely unreliable' to 'only moderately unreliable'. We used to guess where on the A55 road to Wales we would break down. One year we stopped all the holiday traffic by having a wheel fall off on a particularly nasty bend towards Bangor.

School days were easy, once I had overcome my hysterics at being left at nursery school by my mum. Having rarely been separated during my first four or five years I was reluctant in the extreme, initially. This must have been even more fraught for my mother, and for the nursery teacher handling a gangly wriggling little brat. At infant and junior school I felt safe and secure with my teachers and friends, and was certainly never aware of any of the dangers today's youngsters seem to face.

Roads were less congested and, from what I can remember, we were able to play in public places free from danger. Certainly though, some aspects of school life were rather less safe than they are today, particularly the smooth and unyielding concrete the play areas were built on. Great for securing climbing frames, but somewhat harder than the infant skulls that used to bounce off it falling from them.

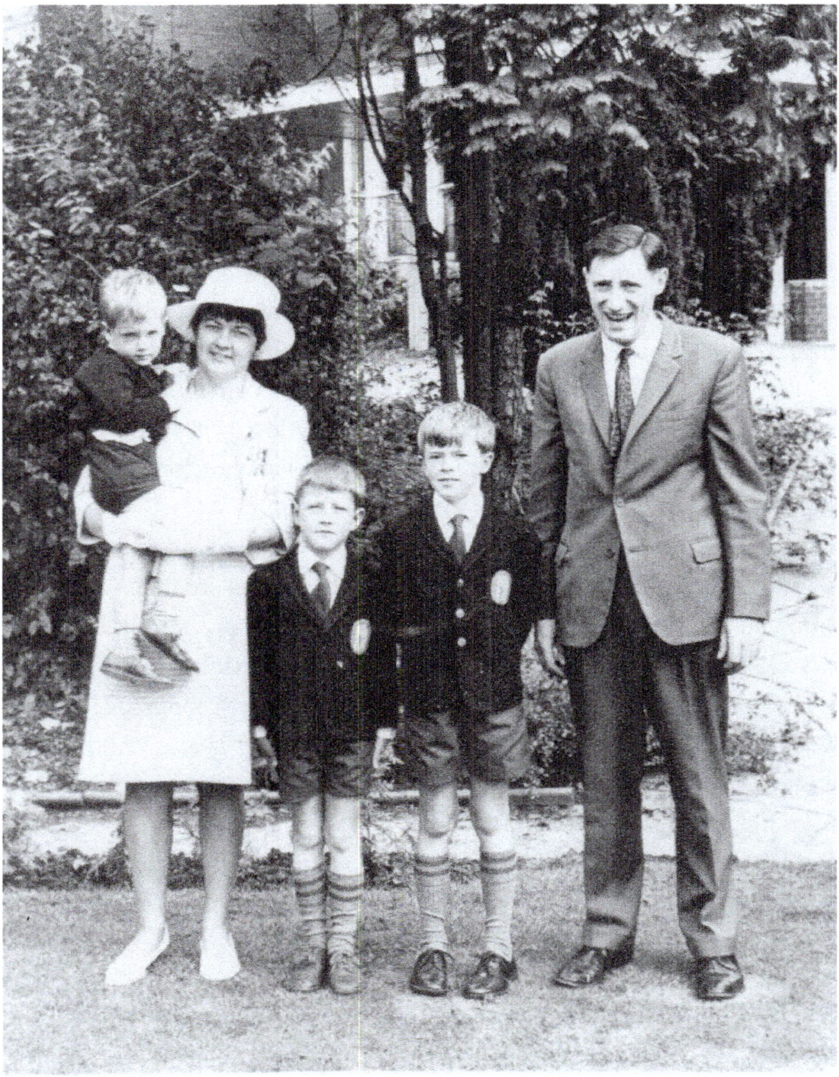

Guy, Mum, Alec, Me and Dad, 1968

I also have a vivid memory of one poor classmate screaming in agony as his hand became caught between the rope climbing-net and the metal crossbar it was draped over, while a dozen children bounded unknowingly up and down the net. It's fortunate the fingers weren't actually severed, as this was before the days of reconstruction microsurgery.

I think I was fortunate enough at junior school to be fairly bright, though any success was not particularly due to trying hard. Dick and Dora's adventures in my reading books sped past fairly rapidly. Nowadays, in my own children's books, Dick and Dora have been replaced by Tom and Sophie, mums seem to work more and dads less, and there is more ethnic awareness – but otherwise not much seems to have changed.

'Impetuous' was how Mrs Wishart, my stern Scottish third-year junior teacher, described me. Unfortunately, even at the age of nine this was pretty accurate, and even more unfortunately for my wife and those around me, this trait has continued. I still have a tendency to feel that if something needs doing, it needs doing immediately.

Marbles, conkers and whether Manchester United were better than Manchester City were my main priorities in my last years at junior school. Those, and winning the sack race for four years running for the Blue Team. Shortly after that, teams seemed to go out of fashion.

I do have some recollections of worrying about the injustices of life at that time, not only regarding myself, for whom there were no real injustices, but others. Most schoolchildren have a cruel streak in them at some time, partly exposed by their peers. Those children not blessed with dexterity and perfect co-ordination, were referred to as 'spazzes' or 'mongs'. This used to worry me even then as, apart from being inaccurate, it was unfair to those who did have cerebral palsy, Down's syndrome or some other disability – not that I understood fully at the time.

I was very pigeon-toed in my early years, and used to fall over my own feet regularly. My chiropodist made me wear hideously big black shoes with built-up soles, and this was before Doc Martens were fashionable. They appeared rather incongruous with my stick legs and knobbly knees. In fact, I looked like a pale version of one of the unfortunate children in famine-stricken Biafra at the time, but wearing shoes belonging to a Disney character!

Through the mists of time I also see an elderly lady with acromegaly (giantism) peddling a bicycle behind a single-decker bus, the back row of which was occupied by schoolchildren pointing at her and laughing hysterically. I felt like crying with her. Not that I was much better. A Scottish classmate of mine, who for some reason wanted to make friends with me, offered me a share of his cakes, to which I replied, 'I dinna wan' any o' ya cakes.' Fortunately we became best friends for many years, until he went to Japan to play professional golf, and after I visited him at the age of 24, I never heard from him again. Perhaps he never really forgave me.

Outside school, I spent the long holidays playing with my friends in various life-threatening situations; narrow fast-flowing streams with rope swings over them, and quarries still being worked, spring to mind. We also turned my parents' garden into a mud bath playing football. We used to bicycle everywhere. Protective wear was not available at the time, and if it had been, we probably would not have worn it as it was not cool. We did, having said that, have lights for our bikes, though the batteries ran out or got wet quickly. I was knocked over at a roundabout by a car, the driver of which didn't see me, partly I think by not being aware of bicycles, but partly because it was dusk and my lights were not on. This has made me very aware of the need to be well illuminated, unlike some of today's youngsters, particularly those on paper rounds who seem to enjoy dicing with death.

Cubs every week at the local church hall was interesting at first, but within a few months I began to realise that while my group spent time picnicking and gardening, other packs seemed to be off mountaineering up the north face of the Eiger, and white-water canoeing. I also had a big problem with knots, which is possibly one of the reasons I did not go in for surgery, so I left fairly soon after joining. Yet another pastime I lost interest in. I did get to attend church most Sundays, where some people also went to pray and practise their Christianity, and others went to show off their new hats, and to see if their neighbours were wearing the same dress as last week. This put me off attending church for many years and has probably unjustifiably affected my views of organised religion.

I was soon to have any illusions about being particularly clever shattered, by failing spectacularly to pass the entrance examinations to Manchester, Stockport and Cheadle Hulme grammar schools. At the latter, I dropped my flask of whatever drink I had, and the fragments of plastic therein distracted my thinking, but I have no excuse whatever for failing the others. Some years later, my father told me that I would have been accepted on a fee-paying reserve place at Stockport, as a patient of his was a school governor, but fortunately we didn't have sufficient funds. I did, however, pass my 'eleven-plus', and so proceeded to Bramhall Grammar School – to become, one year later, Bramhall Comprehensive School. Unfortunately, most of my friends at the time didn't get through this arbitrary selection procedure, and went their own ways to secondary modern schools. I am sure they were at least as bright as I was, but perhaps unlucky on the day, or nervous, or at the age of 10 or 11, not best assessed in an examination situation.

At the end of the 1960s, also the end of my primary education, I had precious little idea what went on in the real world, which at the age of 10 is probably not a bad thing.

We had no videos, nasty or otherwise, and evening television only, which was censored rather more heavily than now. I had little idea about Vietnam, Northern Ireland, South Africa, racial prejudice or poverty. The nearest I could identify to any of it was in having a crew-cut hairstyle which, if the back of my head hadn't stuck out so far, might have made me look like an American astronaut or soldier. Those just a few years older than me had long hair, ridiculous clothes and an appreciation of the Beatles or Jimi Hendrix.

The only time I can remember the television being on in the morning was on the day man first landed on the moon, when we all got up at the crack of dawn, filled with excitement and awe. This, however, was the nearest I would ever get to being an astronaut, and having given up my piano lessons before I reached Grade 1, my musical aspirations were also nonstarters. What would the 1970s and my teens have in store?

CHAPTER TWO

JOSTLE – V.T./I. Push roughly, as my dictionary defined the word. Or – bump, butt, crowd, elbow, hustle, jog, joggle, jolt, press, push, scramble, shake, shove, squeeze, thrust (thesaurus entry).

This was the first word I learned the meaning of as I arrived at the enormous flat-roofed box-like buildings of my secondary school. There was I, minding my own business in a blazer and trousers only moderately too large – and, of course, no cap, as I had heard you got your head flushed down the toilet if you wore one of those – when suddenly the cry went up and hordes of larger youths converged on the passageway between the buildings where I and a few other new boys were cowering. We were carried away, feet several inches off the ground, and squashed against the outer doors, which were still locked from the inside.

Occasionally, the wave of menacing dark-clothed hooligans would ease off, only to wash back again, against the puny driftwood newcomers. If you were lucky almost a whole breath could be taken in between surges. When the doors opened we flowed along the corridors to be deposited in the main hall, where we tried to recover our composure, safe at least in the knowledge that we had survived thus far, and most of the boys were now no bigger than the rest of us, though the girls were at least a foot taller.

A skeletal man with a shiny bald head marched in, gown flowing behind him, followed by several equally serious-looking men and women who were to be our new form teachers. By name, we were divided into classes, and '1H' (for Higginbottom) as we were known, soon trooped off to our new classroom through what seemed like miles of corridor.

Years later, on revisiting the school, the walk seemed like only a few yards, and all the buildings looked so much smaller and less threatening. The gowns had gone, the headmaster had gone. The only thing which hadn't changed was the clouds of cigarette smoke billowing from the teachers' staff room; even that has probably now gone. Perhaps they hide behind the bike sheds for a quick cigarette now, with the pupils.

Mrs Higginbottom was a large friendly lady who made us feel a lot more at ease. This sense of well-being lasted for nearly an hour until we were introduced to our PE teacher in the changing rooms.

Whack! All nervous mutterings stopped completely as this huge muscular bearded man walked around the room after slamming a wooden table-tennis bat, with no foam on, against the gleaming tiles. We were left in no doubt that anyone who even vaguely stepped out of line would have his backside introduced to that bat several times, very hard.

I escaped that punishment, but I very nearly did not escape being one of the last boys in Bramhall High School to be caned, before corporal punishment was abolished. It was my considerable misfortune to be declared form captain, as my name was just about first on the register. One day our teacher was late, and an ink fight broke out among some of the aspiring jostlers in my class. Soon, thanks to these three boys, we and most of the walls were covered in dot-to-dot trails of ink. The three culprits were sent off to the 'beak', along with me who, at the last minute, was slip-roaded into the deputy head's office. There I was told I was lucky not to be in the headmaster's room being caned, as I had not stopped the riot in 'my' class. I tried to protest that the other three were bigger and fiercer than I, but realised I should cut and run as I was shown the door, from where I could hear the yelps of my classmates.

After this baptism of fire, matters settled down somewhat and, as most of us do, I found some new non-ink-throwing friends, and a liking for most of my teachers. The variety of subjects was stimulating, and with my mother to do much of the English homework, including some inspired poetry, and my father to do most of my woodwork and metalwork projects, life was quite easy. How on earth my teachers could reconcile my uninspired classwork with my outstanding homework I'll never know. For instance, out of what seemed to be a 1 metre cubed piece of hardwood I fashioned a 5cm long fish in a whole term of woodwork, yet from home I brought in a scale model replica of a particular lighthouse, fashioned on a lathe and complete with flashing light on top. These projects pulled up my classwork to such an extent that in the first and second year I was near the top in our results table for most subjects. This was encouraging for me, but these tables must have been demoralising for those who were less fortunate.

One totally unexpected area I led the field in was cross-country running. I still remember the first year race vividly. We set off on a cold autumnal day to squelch around a valley for two or three miles before returning to the school. At the bottom of the first hill one of my shoes came off, which I then carried. In spite of this, within a few minutes I found myself way ahead in front of the rest. In fact, I could almost imagine a hint of admiration from the ink-throwers, and as I toiled back up the hill, they finished their cigarettes ready to rejoin the race at a plausible position, having missed out the loop around the valley. When I passed there all these years later, there is still the vague smell of leaking sewers, which I must have gulped in by the litre in my formative years, which still evokes strong memories.

This running ability was a mixed blessing. I enthusiastically joined the cross-country running team, but I was also press-ganged into the rugby team. Although I resembled a stick insect, the fact that I could run apparently made me a promising winger. The other reason was that most of the other boys had more sense. On occasions, seven or eight of us turned up for a Saturday match, much to the embarrassment of our teachers, who would then lecture us at length about school spirit, comradeship and so on. It is, however, not easy to be buoyed up by 'school spirit' when one is bounced unceremoniously over the sideline with a bleeding nose by a boy a foot taller and wider than oneself, with hairy legs and a voice several octaves lower than mine. I think we lost that match 72–0.

What I lacked in testosterone, I tried to make up for in dextrose tablets as I ran twice a week for Manchester Athletics Club, and swam once a week for Stockport Swimming Club. As if all the chauffeuring around by various parents wasn't enough, I also played table tennis on the remaining weekday night, and raced on Saturday mornings.

'This was young Clive Barker's best show to date,' read the back page headline of the *Stockport Advertiser* one winter week in 1971. Shortly after, the Manchester Athletics Club Under-12 team won a national cross-country event, with yours truly coming fourth individually. Any hope of reaching puberty in the next few years was dashed by all these exertions, and as well as a few medals I also collected what seems like one of the most persistent cases of athlete's foot in medical history. Unfortunately, the more I trained, the worse I became in comparison with the other lads and again, like so many things I have taken up in my life, my enthusiasm dwindled and I retired from most competitive sports at the grand old age of 13 or 14.

At that time, my father's dental practice was thriving, sustained by ever-increasing varieties of sugar-loaded foods, and lack of fluoride. Soon the practice overran the house, so that for a short while we all lived upstairs in a small portion of the house, until we were able to move into our new home. This would mean that at last my parents had broken away from living over the shop. Now we were to live over the road from the shop. This was a fairly impressive house called 'White Walls', with seven bedrooms, a big cellar, games room, and a servants' call box in the kitchen. It also had a huge garden, though half of this had to be sold off to a local builder, so we could actually afford to live in this mansion. In fact, my parents had a year of sleepless nights in between buying the house and garden, and selling the lawn, on which two new houses soon stood.

We loved living there, though it was a labour of love. It wasn't designed for those with relatively modest means, hence the games room had an ageing tennis-table table in, instead of a billiards table, and instead of servants we had an occasional cleaning lady who used to leave her false teeth on the work surface in the kitchen. The leaded windows were dreadful to clean, and not very insulating, but as double glazing was too expensive, we had one winter where we had an inside layer of clingfilm over them. This must have appalled the neighbours, some of whom could actually afford to live in these houses.

In fact, we were a small cul-de-sac of four houses, the numbers of which were displayed on a white sign at the entrance of the drive, where someone added 'Burglars Look!' Unfortunately some did, and we were burgled several times, though mainly their hauls consisted of sausages and tomatoes, and the occasional coffee table. On one occasion we were all in the lounge watching *Alias Smith and Jones*, including our springer spaniel, Elsa, when they came in upstairs from the balcony and rifled through my parents' dressing tables. The house did enable my brothers and me to study in relative seclusion, and to play with our friends in safety. In the following years my mum would shout herself hoarse when tea was ready, as we all did our homework with music blaring from separate stereo systems, or with our earphones on.

In the school holidays we went on educational trips. I spent my second year summer holiday learning how lonely I could be in the south of France, staying with a French family for five weeks. This could have been wonderful, but in retrospect I was too young, and too feeble to take advantage of the opportunity. This was not helped by the fact that the girl I was exchanging with, who stayed with us the previous summer, had changed into a stunning young woman. She was rather mismatched with a skinny 13-year-old boy whose 'right on' early seventies hairstyle had him mistaken for a girl by a friend of her family, which sapped any remaining confidence I had. My French was poor, and now the only three phrases I recall from five years schooling in French are: *Je m'appelle Charles* – I am called Charles (this was the nearest we could get in French to Clive); *Non ce n'est pas une regle* – no, it is not a ruler; and *Je voudrais aller a l'universite pour etudier la medicine* – I would like to go to university to study medicine. I was the first in my class to be asked what I would like to do, and it obviously seemed an easy answer, as half the class then said the same, much to the teacher's chagrin. Perhaps I had hankerings after a career in medicine even then, though I was the only pupil who did eventually go directly into medical school following my secondary education.

In the third year, I went on a school cruise around the Mediterranean. Again I was homesick, but this time I was also seasick, and scared stiff! As one of my astute friends at the time said, 'There were several classes of travel on the Nevassa – first, second and third class, and "Colditz style".' We were below the water level, dormitoried with psychopaths from other schools. In Naples, one boy came back on board with a huge knife and another with a gun!

By the fourth year, however, as I gained height and hair, my confidence grew slightly. The German class went youth-hostelling down the great rivers, and this I enjoyed. The 'harder' boys exuded confidence that I could only dream of, though. They would talk assuredly with the female members of our party, and resented any intrusions from the rest of us. What really irritated me, though, was that some of them were younger than me. One moment I remember vividly is sitting eating our gruel, and one of those lads talked at me, and told me my father was his dentist. He said that he was the best dentist from Land's End to John O'Groats. This made me burst with pride, though naturally I was cool enough not to be too acknowledging. If my children could feel as proud as I did then, I would indeed be lucky.

I didn't learn anything on these holidays apart from how other people French-kissed, and smoked foreign cigarettes, and though I was involved in neither of these, I was beginning to enjoy my little adventures abroad.

While I was relieved that I had actually started to grow, it seems to be the elder child's fate to surprise family friends by their progress. I vaguely remember shuffling in an embarrassed manner while people would comment on how grown up I looked. This used to draw parallels for me with a sketch from my favourite TV programme of the time, *Monty Python's Flying Circus*. There, John Cleese, at six-feet six-inches tall, and wearing a business suit and bowler hat, would return home to his mother, where she and a friend were played by two of the other five male Monty Python team.

'Oooh, hasn't he grown!' I remember one cackling. 'And he can talk now!' they exclaimed.

'Yes, of course I can talk,' said an exasperated Cleese. 'I'm minister for overseas development!'

I did start getting down to some work during term time though. I recall I took maths, physics, chemistry, biology, English literature, English language, French and German O levels. History and geography, though good for days out on field trips, I couldn't fit in. Classics the school didn't teach at that level. Religious education was taught by a genial old reverend in such a soporific way he couldn't have stirred any interest had he been teaching the disciples, so that too was dropped. Similarly, I had little talent for practical subjects and art, apart from making pottery models of little Jimmy Osmond and then smashing them to smithereens. We had what was laughingly called human biology/sex education, of which the latter lasted less than one lesson, taught by a biology teacher who was even more embarrassed than we were.

The subjects I did carry on with I enjoyed, apart from setting fire to myself accidentally leaning over a Bunsen burner during a chemistry lesson, which was more upsetting than it was dangerous. The only other time I ended up with the school nurse was when I ran into a door and knocked myself clean out. These days that would be a clear-cut indication for admission via casualty for X-rays and a short period of observation. At that time, once I could walk I was told to go home, approximately a mile's walk, and tell my mum. By the time I staggered up the drive I had a beautiful shiner which, needless to say, caused some consternation.

I began to get a satisfaction from working out and understanding theories and equations, and definitely began to lean towards favouring the sciences by my O-level years. I still had no idea whatsoever regarding career choice, and careers advice from the school was conspicuous by its absence at that stage. However, I kept my options open by opting for maths, physics and chemistry A levels, providing I could get good enough grades at O level. These I was fortunate enough to achieve, and so I was able to pass, via a couple of long hot summers, into my sixth-form studies.

At this stage I, along with the rest of my generation, lost any remaining sense of taste by trying to grow up wearing the most hideous attire of any generation before or since. Disco fever was rife, and I still cringe at memories of myself falling off my platform shoes while trying to dance. I have a photograph of my mother's father holding a lollipop lady's sign which says 'STOP – Children'. No wonder, as beside him I am dressed in a garish blue-and-white checked jacket, black shirt, white kipper tie, and enormous flares, and I have ludicrously long flowing hair. Some months later, I wore this to see my first X-rated film (*M.A.S.H.*) with a male friend, equally badly dressed, as we were under the misguided impression we actually looked 18 years old, when in fact all we looked was ridiculous.

On a more serious note, my father's father was unknowingly giving me an insight into what illness, and more specifically cigarette-smoking induced illness, can do. From being so successful in his middle years, as his arteries began to clog up, so his cerebral function shut down. Within a few years he couldn't recognise his own children, never mind grandchildren. One of my saddest memories is of him at his 70th birthday party, thanking us for attending, 'Though I don't have many words left.' He died not long after, of a heart attack following minor strokes.

The sciences took me out of the fashionable group of pupils doing economics, sociology and law, into a band of rather more serious and certainly more spotty students, who in our spare time would discuss the finer points of rock groups like Genesis and Pink Floyd. At that time few girls were encouraged to study sciences, though maybe they had more sense. Contact with the opposite sex was therefore limited and, having no girlfriends, we had lots of time to listen to music, and to work, which I had to do increasing amounts of. This was because, while O levels had come naturally, I did not have the kind of brain which adjusted easily to pure and applied mathematics. This I found deeply frustrating, and perhaps I drifted from pure science towards my eventual career.

Looking back through my old diaries, which I have kept since 1976, more as a forward planner and organiser than a record of events, I am struck by how much swotting I used to do. This wasn't out of desire, but necessity. I also seemed to have spent almost as much time planning my revision as doing it!

As a break from book work I tried to branch out at weekends and in the evenings with one or two of my more outgoing friends, and I started going to the local youth club. As I could play table tennis and tennis I met new friends and even some girls. Becoming braver, I auditioned for parts in productions at school of *The Pirates of Penzance* and *Patience,* and since no one was ever turned away, I became a heavy dragoon and other unlikely characters.

One character I wasn't planning to be up to this time was a doctor, but it was time to choose which route in my working life I was to take. Careers advice was still scant. Dentistry didn't appeal to me. In medicine one explores more bizarre areas than the mouth, but at least they vary. Five years at university appealed to me though, and as I couldn't think of anything else to do I chose medicine. I would like to think, twenty years later, that at the risk of sounding pretentious, medicine chose me, as I am sure I couldn't have picked a more suited vocation to what I wanted to put in to, and get out of, life.

We therefore filled in our university application forms. For a subject like medicine, where an ability to communicate is important, I found it surprising that some universities did not hold interviews. Manchester had recently changed buildings, and become the biggest medical school in Europe. Quite why that attracted me I am not sure, but I applied and was accepted, provided I got the needed 'three Bs'. This I duly did, and thus put off the day I would actually have to work for a living, until the age of 23.

I thoroughly enjoyed that final long end-of-school holiday, though I had to spend the first few days of it in bed. This was because at the end of the exams, a couple of teachers and several pupils, now of age, had gone to a local pub to celebrate. Having not been used to drinking large volumes of beer, I consumed several pints, which I then deposited along with the rest of my stomach contents over the bed, my bedroom floor, the landing, and my parents' room, as I staggered in around midnight saying, 'I think I've been ill.' Fortunately, Mum and Dad were sympathetic enough to put this down to experience, lay me in the recovery position after cleaning me up, and checked I was still in fact alive from time to time. Though I felt ashamed about this, I understand my physics teacher was even more embarrassed, as he was last reported walking off in the other direction with a toilet seat around his head.

I recall another of my schoolfriends, who sadly I lost contact with some years ago, making me realise that we were on the verge of an unknown future, and that the relative security of school days was over. As we said our goodbyes with our exam results in our hands, he wished me well saying, 'Have a good life.'

CHAPTER THREE

I was invited to look around two medical schools other than Manchester. Leeds looked even more like a concrete jungle, though Leicester was rather more personal and actually did hold interviews. I understand my references had been reasonable, though even at that stage my head teacher's main concern was whether I would be able to 'wind down' from the concerns of a working day in medicine, and to relax. However, I plumped for Manchester, and having arrived early at nearly every destination in my life (a habit I hope to break before my death), I reached the enormous medical school on my first morning nearly an hour early. This gave me time to wander up and down Oxford Road, feeling increasingly nervous and insecure. Eventually, I plucked up courage to enter the dark, sparsely windowed building, and walked silently towards the notice board where the names of the first year students were displayed.

I wasn't on the list. In alphabetical order there were only two Barkers, an Olive Barker and a Sue Barker. My heart sank. Had I not been accepted after all? Was I looking at the wrong list? Then my heart sank even further. How many 18-year-old Olives were there in the late 1970s? Though it had never happened before, the awful realisation dawned that Clive is written in exactly the same way as Olive, only with a millimetre or two less type separating the ends of the C. Later that morning my worst fears were confirmed. A typing error had entered me for five years of medical school as Olive Barker. Thus I was known to many of my friends and some of my lecturers throughout the coming terms.

Other anxious acne-ridden 18-year-olds gradually gathered around the board, and then along with them I walked apprehensively and dejectedly up to the first floor where the main lecture theatre was situated. We filed in and dispersed up the 15 or so rows of tiered seats. Some people were actually talking to each other. Why hadn't I got any friends yet? The previous evening I had attended a 'freshers' disco' in the Union bar, another dark and this time subterranean room which smelled of stale smoke, stale beer and stale students. I had made one or two medical and non-medical contacts, and fortunately another lad and I recognised each other the following morning and chatted amiably in the lecture theatre.

At 18 years old I was getting better at starting school all over again. By a complete fluke, I was to have sitting on my other side two likeable chaps who introduced themselves. One of them, on hearing my name was Clive, raptured into a fair impression of 'Clive Jenkins of the trade union movement', in an authentic Welsh accent. He, I decided, was either being rude, or just being extrovertly friendly. I judged the latter, which is just as well, as 11 years later Ewan was to be my best man. His friend Graham and I also remain firm friends all these years later. They had an advantage over me in that they lived in halls, and thus had met a couple of days before. I was to become an honorary member of their hall, and got to know their carpets intimately as I crashed out on various floors in the coming two years.

On our first day we had a series of introductory lectures from various members of staff. The only fact I remember was, I think, from a professor of medicine, who told us that statistically one of the two hundred of us would be dead before the course was up.

We came from all sorts of backgrounds: from comprehensive schools like mine, to some of the more renowned public schools – though more were to join from these in our third year, from St Andrew's University. Many nationalities were represented, and yet again I had chosen a course predominantly peopled by men, though in recent years the numbers have equalised. Interestingly, not many of the students' parents were doctors. There was a wide spectrum of characters too. A few seemed socially completely ill at ease, which reinforced my belief in the need for interviews for medicine. Mainly they had taken maths, further maths, and even more maths for A level, and chemistry, which enabled them to do medicine. To communicate on any level other than advanced mathematics theory seemed impossible, and how such people were to communicate with patients I don't know!

There were a few confident rugger types, but fortunately not too many who were there by virtue of who their parents knew. Mostly, my compatriots were relatively normal, at that stage at least.

I, and my new-found acquaintances, trooped off around the university to view the stalls laid out in various buildings for freshers' week. Manchester University is not based on a campus. It is a series of mainly grey buildings, at either side of an equally grey main road, under a grey sky. Having recently walked the Pennine Way with my family, I joined the hiking club. I wasn't confident enough at that stage to join any others, but my contemporaries in halls were kind enough to invite me to be thrashed on their squash courts a few times. I fell in with a nice crowd and soon realised that they had been as nervous as I had, and they had probably more reason to be, as most were living away from home for the first time. I couldn't qualify for a living away grant, as my home was eight miles from the university, and we couldn't afford to fund living in halls, so I commuted from home. This was either by bus, train, bicycle (which I doubt I would do now), or by a series of small cars of varying degrees of unreliability. For a brief period in my pubertal years, I was probably a pain to my parents and brothers, but by the age of 18 I knew I was on to a good thing and we all got on well.

All we medical students had one thing in common. We were all going to become doctors, apart from a handful who decided to leave, and an even smaller handful who were to fail, a feat which was pretty difficult, though we didn't know it at the time. If the Government was going to spend £55,000, at late 1970s costings, on training each medical student over five years, it wasn't too impressed if there were many failures. We all sat from nine thirty in the morning to about four thirty in the afternoon being lectured at, many frantically taking notes in the hope that facts would stick more firmly than if they were gleaned only out of the vast amount of text books we also bought. We digested huge amounts of information, most of which we have never used since. A few lectures were interesting, many were mediocre, and quite a few were mind-numbingly boring. Several were so confusing that they set me back months. I particularly remember a physiology lecture about cell membranes, in which each feature was represented as a vegetable. A novel idea perhaps, but I, and several others, were obviously missing the relevant lobe of brain necessary to comprehend this – or perhaps the lecturer was.

One worry early on was how we would cope with what was for

most of us our first sight of a dead body. This was not as harrowing as anticipated, as the subjects in question had been prepared and preserved so that they looked so unlifelike that it was hard to imagine they had ever been alive … so pale, cold and waxy. We settled down to anatomy, physiology, biochemistry and countless more subjects with enthusiasm, taking an exam at the end of each term on what we had covered, and then forgetting most of it forever.

In the seven months we were actually there, for each of the first two years, we packed quite a lot of other activities in too. Wednesday afternoons were always free, for sport. I was so put off by the seemingly international standards required, that with some of my friends sport consisted of a pub lunch of bread and cheese and a suitable hand-pulled ale which combined to give one a wonderful sense of well-being, and flatulence! I didn't drink excessively as I was often driving, when my parents could lend me the car, and even then a lot depended on whether the car I used was working. What little I know about car maintenance, I have learned from figuring out which part of the ailing cars I was driving had conked out, at any given time. Triumph Toledos were almost manageable, but for a short while I had the mixed fortune to drive a Vauxhall Viva. I know, as most driving students do, how Basil Fawlty felt when thrashing his car with a branch, as it broke down at all sorts of inconvenient times, including on the morning of my second term exams. The garage from which we bought this car seemed to have a 'timeshare' agreement, where we had it for one week and they had it for one week, alternating for the few months until we gave it back to them!

On more than one occasion it broke down after an evening with my first girlfriend at university, honestly. She and I met on a parachuting weekend, and as the weather was too wet and windy to parachute we spent quite a lot of time together. She was a year older than I, and seemingly more worldly wise, with virtually no inhibitions. Late one cold winter night, when I phoned my parents to say I couldn't get home, and reassured them I was sure her parents wouldn't mind me staying there, my virginity was lost all too quickly. I should have known I was in out of my depth, figuratively speaking, when she presented me with a book of sexual positions, open at the description of the big toe as an erogenous zone. Since I scarcely knew what to do with my penis, never mind my toe, I felt matters were progressing rather too quickly. Some years later I did complete a parachute jump, and found it considerably less scary, and more exhilarating, than those earlier experiences.

My first Easter holiday at university, I spent with three other men, possibly as a reaction to what had happened shortly before, partaking in an experiment run by the medical school. This involved being locked in an isolation unit, with four layers of walls and no windows between the one room we occupied, with en-suite toilet and shower, and the outside world. No light, sound or anything from the real world could get in, apart from the chap running the experiment who delivered our food every three days or so. Inside, our waking and sleep times were mixed up, split up, and generally messed up, until we had no idea what time of day or night it was. Our bodily functions were monitored, in particular urine output and temperature, to see if they corresponded with how awful we felt. We must have been desperate for money, for we did all this for £50 for two weeks. Not bad in the late 1970s for students perhaps, until one considers the temperature was taken with continuous monitoring by rectal thermometer. At night we plugged the other end of this wire leading from our bottoms into a bedside socket. This presented a major problem when one of us forgot to unplug himself before jumping off the top bunk! What is really worrying, however, is that we all did it again the following Easter, though for the huge sum of £85.

I remember soulfully listening to an Elton John record on the tinny stereo we had, missing a girl I was trying to court, as Elton sang 'What have I got to do to make you want me?' The answer was probably not to spend two weeks with a thermometer up my bottom, in the company of three other men, competing for who had the most offensive body odour by the end of the two weeks. While doing nothing for my love life, I am sure this experience set me even more permanently on the path of heterosexuality.

Some of our fellow students had other ways of earning a few pounds. One of the other bizarre ways for which male medical students were chosen, was sperm donation. This gave a whole new meaning to the phrase 'being hard up', and I understand some of my year did make a few deposits in the sperm bank. This is, of course, an important and helpful way of aiding some couples with fertility problems. Some of my less charitable friends suggested that one of our number earned so much money from masturbation at university, his forearms were as muscular as Popeye's!

I tried taxing my body in other ways, and attempted the infamous Bogle stroll sponsored walk in rag week. This is a 55-mile trek from Manchester to Wigan and Chorley and back again. What a pointless exercise! The first time I ever visited Chorley was at about seven o'clock on a rainy morning, having walked there from Manchester. Perhaps it exerted some kind of gravitational pull on me, as when I tried to leave it to head back to Manchester I started seizing up. By the time I had reached Walkden further down the A6, after 47 miles, little old ladies with walking sticks (and I think I even recall one with a frame, though I may have been hallucinating by that stage) were overtaking me. As I ground to a halt I remember seeing a young lad standing in a puddle in the rain, and thinking, 'How stupid!' Then I thought of myself, a supposedly intelligent young man wearing a non-waterproof tracksuit, spending 13 hours nearly killing myself by walking around in a big circle. Perhaps he was not the stupid one. Next year I managed it, though I retired from long-distance walking forever after that.

The only lasting harm I did my body in that first year was on a beach in Blackpool in the summer term. After a fish-and-chips and beer lunch, my so-called friends decided to bury me in the sand. Foolishly I struggled, sending a searing pain through my left arm. Having not yet completed the upper limb in anatomy, I shouted that I had dislocated my elbow and, this obviously not being the case, my colleagues continued to bury me. Shortly after I must have changed colour, as they then did stop to observe my shoulder not being the same shape as it was before. Having finally twigged that my shoulder was dislocated, a policeman was located – not, unfortunately, to arrest those who had got me into this situation, but to summon an ambulance. I knelt on the promenade in sheer agony while elderly ladies tottered by looking with interest as if I was some kind of tourist attraction. In fact, I am sure one of them had previously overtaken me on my sponsored walk some months earlier.

What followed was my only experience as a patient on an ambulance journey. This was unbelievably bumpy, but the experience was relieved slightly by some nitrous oxide gas. Five hours later, when my lunch had settled, under a short general anaesthetic my shoulder was relocated. This meant that I travelled everywhere for a while by bus or train. On one evening, my boarding station was unmanned and on arrival in Manchester I tried a rather stupid prank, by saying I had boarded two stations later than I in fact had, which would have saved me about 20p. Of course I got found out and was fined. I worried so much about this that I have been obsessively honest ever since.

A week before my first year exams I unexpectedly found myself spending four days in Montreal, Canada. My Scottish schoolfriend, Iain, had been given two complimentary airline tickets by his father for the inaugural jumbo jet service from Manchester to Montreal. In fact, it was his father who was originally offered the tickets but due to other working commitments, which involved him travelling far and wide, he couldn't make it.

In spite of the testing academic time ahead, I couldn't resist going when invited. Hence we found ourselves at the departure lounge of Manchester Airport VIP Suite eating cucumber sandwiches and drinking champagne, looking somewhat out of place with the businessmen who surrounded us. We had an excellent four days, and calmly boarded the hotel bus to the airport for our return journey in good time. Arriving at check-in we were aghast to find that there were two airports in Montreal, and we had arrived at the wrong one. Virtually penniless, and with no time left to spare, we somehow crossed the city courtesy of a charitable taxi driver in record time to board our correct plane from the correct airport. For a moment though, I had seen my medical career evaporate.

At the end of the academic year, exams duly taken and hopefully passed, we set about seriously partying. In fact, we looked seriously daft dancing badly to songs from *Saturday Night Fever* and *Grease*. I also attended my first music festival, when four friends and I drove down to Knebworth Park to see Genesis from a long way away. In our excitement to get within earshot of the stage, on arrival we abandoned the car and headed to the arena. Our problems began when the concert ended and we discovered there were 40 acres of car parking space for one hundred thousand people and we had no idea where we had left my car. A frantic hour later we found it. We then had plenty of time to relax as it took three hours to get out of the car park. The tiredness I felt then was a little insight into that which I was to feel in my working years ahead.

Holiday work was hard to come by; having been turned down by McVitie's Biscuits, to whom I had applied as I was tempted by the delicious ginger or digestive aroma as I cycled past in the mornings, I signed on the dole. This was a demoralising experience that I've been lucky enough never to have had to do since. After a short while I signed off again, to set off on a shoestring-budgeted trip with two university friends around Europe. We covered six thousand miles, thirteen countries and hundreds of yards of toilet roll, in five weeks. Living on mushroom omelette and camaraderie, my weight dropped to under ten stones which, for my six-foot frame, left me almost as skeletal as in my prepubertal years. In fact, one of our little group never recovered, and after flying his hang-glider some months later into Winter Hill transmission tower, left medical school forever.

Most of us found the second year tedious. The lectures were repetitive, uninspiring, and seemingly as unenthusiastically presented as they were received. Real patients seemed as far away as ever, fortunately for them, and the relevance of what we were studying seemed remote. Social events continued, however, and trying to look like we imagined real doctors might, we continued the tradition of winter and summer balls. To my first ball, I invited a young lady in my year who, to my surprise, accepted. Attired in my dinner jacket, I thought I looked rather smart. Unfortunately, the evening before, a small spot appeared on my face which, within 24 hours, had enlarged into a massive boil, which detracted somewhat from the effect. I am not sure why these things always occur when one is trying to impress. Other than that, my first medical ball went swimmingly well, and I even succeeded in a goodnight kiss without direct contact with my facial abscess.

I should have known better than to try to impress. Later that year my then girlfriend (to whom I hadn't exposed any carbuncles) and I spent an illicit couple of days at my parents' home while they were away on holiday. We crept around the house deftly drawing curtains and dimming lights, and were really relaxed when the doorbell was rung by two police officers. I hurtled down the stairs, then back up again, as I realised I had been trying to put my girlfriend's blouse on instead of my shirt. Back downstairs, I tried to persuade them that I was in fact the owner's eldest son and, after a few wry smiles, they departed convinced and I breathed a huge sigh of relief, only to realise that my flies were gaping rather obviously.

At 'work', I planned my revision in increasing detail, and exams came and went. Fortunately, I had more success with those than I did in my love life at that stage, and after another relatively idle summer holiday, we entered the third year and clinical medicine.

CHAPTER FOUR

With dazzling white coats straight out of advertisements for washing powder, we ventured nervously on to the hospital wards at last. We couldn't have looked more conspicuously wet behind the ears if we had tried, and all the doctors, nurses and patients peered dismissively past us. The patients were, in fact, the most pleasant, followed by the junior doctors who vaguely remembered how we were feeling, and least welcoming initially were the nurses. This is hardly surprising, as hordes of medical students were allocated to each ward in these Manchester teaching hospitals.

Our only apparent functions were to ask inane questions and get in the way. The student nurses were somewhat more empathetic, the junior qualified nurses mildly amused, and the senior nurses intimidating. Perhaps they knew that only too soon some of us would get delusions of grandeur, and try to play doctors far too soon. A few of our number were, in fact, embarrassingly pompous just because they knew the course of every irrelevant nerve and blood vessel in the human body. They usually came down to earth fairly quickly when faced with a real patient who knew vastly more about their illness than the student did. Within a short time, we learned that nurses were in fact our most helpful allies, and those of us who recognised our shortcomings and asked for help usually got it.

The senior doctors varied in their attitudes. Some were benign, almost fatherly figures; some were so busy we didn't get to know them well; and some we got to know only too well because they were thoroughly unpleasant and seemed to derive pleasure from embarrassing us in front of our peers, the nurses, doctors, and patients. Admittedly, this was easy as we knew very little about bedside manner, appropriate examination, and practical medicine.

Woe betide any patient who was unlucky enough to have a heart murmur, a palpable liver, or a lump anywhere, as they were auscultated, percussed, and palpated, until they were sick of the sight of anything in a white coat. They were incredibly stoical and seemed to accept that this was part of the privilege of being treated in a teaching hospital. On leaving our half days on the wards, we would shed our serious expressions and go back to being real university students, slovenly and dishevelled.

At this time I moved into a tiny terraced house in Rusholme, Manchester with my two friends from the first days, and Danny, who had met the others on a waterborne pub crawl they called a canal holiday. I had met Danny on a midnight hike up Pendle Hill, where the custom was to sing 'Jerusalem' very badly, on reaching the summit. I tried to take a photograph of us all, and as I was readying the camera, the instamatic flash bulb went off two inches from my widely dilated pupils. I couldn't see a thing for most of the rest of the night. Danny was treasurer of the Manchester University Morris Dancing Society, until it went bankrupt, and he is now in general practice three miles down the road

Our own home was a great adventure for us, knowing we could play at being independent, until our clothes ran out and we could take our washing home. In this house the floors sloped, though the slugs seemed to cope well, as we could see their trails each morning. The walls between the rooms were about as thick as a layer of toilet tissue, so we could hear each other's breathing and other bodily functions. Most of the time it was freezing, and in winter we would huddle around the gas cooker in the morning to warm up. We had a cleaning rota, which disappeared after the third week of our occupancy, so washing up was only done when we had nothing to eat off, and at times we didn't even let that bother us.

Around our home were other students, as well as a large Asian population, some of whom now run excellent restaurants, and an Irish population who run excellent pubs. Ideal student life, in fact. There was a corner shop literally open all hours, though the proprietor's English wasn't too good. Canned food was easy enough but when one of our contemporaries tried to ask for tampons, the partly spoken and partly gestured conversation went on most of the day.

At this time at Manchester University were a group of students who later went on to be *The Young Ones* in the television series about torrid university life. I think we fitted into this scenario quite well. Probably the greatest health hazard we encountered during that year was a café, frequented by students as it was so cheap, where there was only one dish available. This was a chicken biryani. It came in five strengths: mild, medium, hot, suicide, or killer. I once managed a medium, and even then had to drink the water that went with it with both my lips inside the glass to cool off, and became cognisant of the meaning of the expression 'both ends burning'. I think it closed down some years later, probably to the relief of the local canine population, as I am not sure that chicken was an accurate description of what we were eating.

After a term's general medicine, which I quite enjoyed the novelty of, we spent a term in general surgery. We felt surplus to requirements on the medical wards, but the operating theatre took this feeling to new heights. We tried not to get too near to the patient for fear of being asked something too intricate or, worse, standing on the diathermy peddle and incinerating the subject or the surgeon. We therefore stood behind those immediately involved, and peered over so as to stand out as surplus to requirements even more noticeably, occasionally nearly falling forward into the surgeon or nurse, or patient's abdomen.

We learned by trial and error how to approach and communicate with patients. I believe that nowadays more emphasis is given at an early stage to the importance of consultation dynamics. This has to be a good thing, as I am sure that in those days we all asked some crass and insensitive questions, which were treated with more dignity by the patients than we deserved. The medical profession has also learned to be more understanding of people's concerns and hopefully don't discuss someone's condition across that person's bed as if they were an object not involved in decisions regarding their management.

During this year we were joined by 75 students from St Andrew's University in Scotland, who had spent three years in pre-clinical work. They seemed to be somewhat more mature both in years and financially, and were instrumental in organising some excellent social events. They seemed to live in slightly less squalid accommodation than we Mancunians. As a general rule the nearer you got to Manchester city centre the worse the flats became.

Some of the friends we made from north of the border lived in positive luxury in Withington and Didsbury, in imposing shared houses. I understand this meant that at times people would share with others they didn't know too well. This could, of course, lead to teething problems, literally. One of our year wondered why the flat toothpaste tasted so strange, until she realised that she was in fact cleaning her teeth with their new flatmate's spermicidal gel! Not surprisingly, some tenants would move in and then move out again fairly quickly. Fortunately, in our house we all got on remarkably well, and only once fell out when Graham, tired of the washing up not being done, deposited it in Danny's bed!

Our next experience of sleep deprivation was on a youth-hostelling holiday that summer. At our first stop away from it all, over the border, I was insulted by the warden for being from Bramhall: 'Daddy's got a yacht and sister's got a horse, I suppose.' I protested that I hadn't even got a sister, but we were shown to our dormitory and ordered to our bunks. These were so fragile that Ewan swore his bunk creaked every time his heart valves opened and shut that night.

The dormitory was full of people who must have had chronic bronchitis or nasal polyps, as everyone snored – except us as we couldn't sleep. The second night we were overrun by a French school who tried to seek revenge for Agincourt by talking all night. On the third night I was just about to doze off at last, when a youngster with a spinal brace fell out of the top bunk and cried all night, poor lad. However, we were perked up by catching a grouse near the Balmoral estate just before 'the glorious twelfth'. It got caught in our roof rack. We gibletted it with a plastic spoon, and while the rest of the hostel that night ate their Vesta curries, we dined ceremoniously on our catch. Had it been larger than a sparrow, it might actually have been worth it.

CHAPTER FIVE

Our fourth year was entirely clinical and was spent away from university for most of the time. Those cleverer students who were already hankering after teaching hospital careers, secured attachments in the large city hospitals on units they would aspire to work on once they had qualified. We four headed almost as far as we were allowed to stray to get more practical hands-on experience rather than esoterica, we explained. We spent five months in Wrexham, North Wales, but found that the same hierarchies existed, though people had more individual identities, sometimes bordering on the eccentric.

Determined to give surgery a fair chance, I crept into the operating theatre on my first morning, where my consultant had started his list and I grovellingly introduced myself.

'Right, Barker, what's this doing?' the consultant barked, pointing to a mass of someone's insides. I had absolutely no idea what he was talking about, as he jabbed a finger at a thin tube of tissue in our subject's abdomen. I opined that I hadn't a clue.

'Well, it's vermiculating, isn't it?'

'If you say so, sir, then I am sure it is.'

'What does that mean, Barker?'

'No idea, sir.'

'Wormlike! Good God boy! Didn't you do Latin?'

'No, sir.'

From that moment our relationship was doomed. He was old-school and was determined I would learn something even if it meant me being humiliated repeatedly. It was insisted on that I examine every single patient completely, so as to get to know what was normal and what was abnormal. I rather felt this behaviour was itself abnormal as it also involved humiliating the patients, as I poked and prodded every poor soul in their entirety no matter how trivial a procedure they had come in for. I was and still am amazed these patients let me do it.

My friends often had equally bizarre experiences. Danny was attached to a team which specialised in mechanical aids for surgery. At least this meant he wasn't spending two hours straining on retractors, pulling an overweight patient's abdominal walls out of the way. This was of course before the days of laparoscopic keyhole surgery. However, his consultant asked him whether, with the name of Danny, he was Irish and, if so, was he a member of the IRA? If so, poor Danny was informed, the consultant would have to shoot him as he was in the Territorial Army.

After nine weeks of surgery, I spent two weeks in general practice which was, for me, literally a breath of fresh air. To be outside during daylight hours on those crisp winter mornings was a revelation, compared to the stuffy operating theatre atmosphere. To be talked to, rather than at, and to see the patients as people was wonderful. Admittedly, there is a limit to what one can learn observing consultations at that stage of one's medical training, but I thoroughly enjoyed the change.

I was the only one of the four of us who had use of a car, which meant we could get around, but when I went to see my girlfriend at the time back in Manchester, my compatriots were rather stranded where we lived for the first five weeks, at a soon-to-shut-down hospital for the elderly. With their transport gone they spent weekends watching cows defecating in the countryside around this isolated spot. It was therefore flattering for me to be requested to stay with my mates on our weekends off, though I think this was partly for my wheels.

We spent a week in community medicine, the high point of which was going to a low point of several hundred feet down one of the few remaining working mines. That was a real eye-opener, and seeing the conditions at the coalface was a sobering experience, compared to my cushy existence.

Following this, we spent a few weeks in general medicine, which was fairly quiet at the time, and consisted mainly of eating up to three large stodgy hospital meals per day, leading to excessive weight gain, and probably furring up of our circulatory systems.

Back in Manchester, we spent another nine weeks on the city outskirts studying psychiatry. This was challenging, as we had only just begun to master establishing a rapport with patients who weren't experiencing psychological difficulties, at least until they had met us anyway. The other challenge was telling the staff from the patients, as the atmosphere was, by necessity, somewhat informal. Occasionally we students would be mistaken for nurses or doctors, but our self-congratulation was short-lived when we were expected to expedite the mistaken patient's treatment, or discharge them home, at which point our feeling of impotence returned. As students, this was one of the most frustrating aspects. Apart from taking blood or running errands we couldn't actually do very much to help.

However, this feeling changed dramatically in our next attachment which was obstetrics and gynaecology, in the highest of high-tech units in Manchester. Wall-to-wall machines with flashing lights and high-pitched beeps surrounded a floodlit patient, who I initially thought must be undergoing some fantastically new and advanced procedure; but no, she was having a baby. My obstetric training must have been at the high point of unnatural childbirth. Being a 'centre of excellence', the maternity unit did have more than its fair share of complicated pregnancies, so the excessive technology was partly understandable, but 15 years later the balance has swung back to more sensible proportions, or possibly even too far.

Again, the patients were in great demand by medical students, and this time by student midwives too. The senior midwifery sisters were a power to be reckoned with. Not surprisingly, they wanted their midwives to experience and assist as many deliveries as possible, but this made for constant competition, between us and them. All the medical students were expected to deliver 10 babies in our attachment. Impetuous as ever, I was determined to make a good start. On my initial weekend on call I realised for the first time what real sleep deprivation felt like. On Saturday morning I began monitoring a nice lady, who was inconsiderate enough to spend 20 hours in labour, before needing a forceps delivery which, of course, I could not do. I was fortunate enough to be allocated another lady straight away who, after another 20 hours, had an emergency caesarean section. When told she was to have this, she was naturally upset, but not as upset as I was. I concluded that no babies were actually born naturally, at least not when I was around.

By the end of my weeks there, however, by sheer persistence, I did assist more than my required number eventually. During this time I was lucky to be so close to the wonder of childbirth, and to the mental and physical strength of the mothers of those children.

At that time the midwives were less involved in suturing episiotomies than they are now. Thus for every delivery of a baby at which I helped, I sutured at least three ladies' nether regions. Most medical students had done very little suturing before their obstetrics and gynaecology jobs, and it struck me as bizarre that this was often our first significant training.

The frontiers of neonatal intensive care were being redrawn during this time, and occasionally tiny babies would be born at 28-weeks gestation, or even earlier, and be transferred to an even more high-tech world on the floor below. There were strange species of doctors working in these places, for over a 100 hours a week, rarely seeing the outside world, whose skin colour was the same as the cadavers we used to dissect. At that time I realised just what constant pressure and ridiculous hours could do to someone, never mind the patients in their care.

My last attachment that year was nine weeks in summer in a more representative paediatric unit, where the babies weighed at least a few pounds, and the older patients were adolescent. I thoroughly enjoyed this period, perhaps as the children were on my wavelength. If I hadn't followed a career in general practice I would like to think I could have continued in paediatrics. The doctors and nurses almost seemed normal too. In that strange summer of 1981, when parts of England were torn by riots, my friends and I continued in that unreal world that was medical training, making the most of what we were beginning to realise was the last few months before we entered the reality of final examinations and work.

CHAPTER SIX

Some months earlier we had been asked to submit applications for an 'elective period' where each student could spread his or her own wings and study, in the loosest possible sense, for eight weeks, wherever in the world they chose, within reason. If we could convince the medical school administrators that we would gain unique experience which could not be acquired in our standard studies otherwise, we could virtually do anything.

The most studious, career-minded, or broke, stayed in the UK. Some self-sacrificing souls went to various regions of the less developed world, and no doubt gained great experience and great maturity, as well as great bowel upsets and interesting diseases that the more selfish like me missed out on. Some others went to the Caribbean, America and a few to mainland Australia, and one, that is myself, to Tasmania.

My father, when in his National Service, worked with a doctor who following this went via Africa and Queensland to Tasmania, where he became a general medical practitioner, with a passing interest in sheep farming – or was it the other way around? As I knew no other far-flung medical practitioners, and Australians have a reputation for having a good time, I contacted him, and he kindly arranged six weeks in Launceston General Hospital, and two weeks with him.

The plane fare came to £614, more than I had in the world, and again I scrounged from my parents, whose interest-free loan during my student years kept me afloat, or in this case airborne, and off I went. After the debacle in Canada, I was not going to be caught out again. I arrived by train at the airport eight hours early for my flight. Long gone were the days of homesickness, and I strolled excitedly around the city that is Heathrow Airport.

Relieved I had actually arrived at my correct port of embarkation, I settled into the bar, and by the time my flight was called I felt splendid. Chatting up the other passengers, I was offered a place to stay in Sydney before I had even left the departure lounge. On board, things got even better: free drinks before, during and after each meal, of which there were five in twenty hours. Determined to get my money's worth, I accepted their hospitality and was positively euphoric by the time we reached Bombay to refuel. Sobered briefly by the apparent conditions we flew over near Bombay Airport, we then journeyed on to Perth.

Even more disorientated in time than my isolation unit experience, I became focussed very suddenly by the request over the public address system for a doctor to make themselves known to the cabin crew. No one seemed to respond, and the call came again. Though hardly qualified, and hardly coherent, I thought that a final year student was better than no one. The cabin crew felt differently, as when I tottered up to their rest area and offered my limited and not-yet-qualified services, they had a brief conference behind the curtain, before appearing and firmly declining my offer. I was left to dejectedly but relievedly return to my seat, clambering yet again over the stoical elderly lady who had the misfortune to sit between my seat and the aisle which led me frequently to the toilets. By the time I arrived in Tasmania I was unsure whether I had jet lag or a massive hangover, and regretted those pre-breakfast gin and tonics.

A day or two later, almost sobered up, I entered Launceston General Hospital student accommodation, over 10,000 miles from home, to find myself watching the royal wedding of Charles and Diana. So much for getting away from England.

My hospital weeks were an education in everything but medicine. As my consultant agreed, I didn't travel halfway around the world to sit in a hospital. I spent my time playing squash, swimming, and spotlighting. The latter is hunting in the dark with huge battery-powered spotlights, for rabbits, wallabies and other wildlife, some of which I had only previously seen on *Skippy the Bush Kangaroo*.

Also standing out, frighteningly, in my mind is flying in a light aircraft to tiny little islands with a runway consisting of a field with two parallel lines of white markers, in a plane piloted by a man who still seemed to think he was in World War II. We also had plenty of beach barbecues, even though it was winter, and I learned plenty about sheep farming and lambing, making this a varied and, in the main, enjoyable time of 'study'.

After this holiday in Tasmania, I set out for two weeks holidaying in Canbera then Sydney. Canberra was a bizarre sterile place where everyone was either a government official or a student taking soft drugs. Sydney, however, was a wonderfully cosmopolitan city, which I have not found anywhere to better. Perhaps it has become more popular since, but lazy warm spring days in the sun on Bondai beach, followed by strolls around the older areas and harbour were idyllic. Apart from being almost forced into a sex club by a bouncer who thought that in my shorts, map and camera I was easy target in King's Cross, I found everyone wonderfully friendly.

I left Sydney with 21 Australian cents, the equivalent of 13 pence, a daunting feeling all that way from home, but luckily, again, all the drinks on the way home were free too, and this time when a doctor was requested, a suitably earnest and mature chap with a beard stood up immediately and walked soberly to assist.

CHAPTER SEVEN

And so to swotting as I had never swotted before. I spent hours, if not days, planning my revision timetable, which I stuck to rigidly. Book work was becoming increasingly tedious, and to relieve the boredom, and to shut out the dogs and, occasionally, neighbours fighting in the street, I always revised with my earphones on. I probably know more about the works of Supertramp and the Eagles than I did about the workings of the cardiovascular system.

Our tutors were almost as desperate for us to pass as we were. We had hundreds of revision lectures, tutorials, and clinical group discussions. We were lucky enough to have an unassuming senior registrar to teach us for six sessions in the first term on clinical examination. We learned so much from him, that we didn't tell him there were only supposed to be those half dozen meetings, and he carried on all year, in his own time, unknowingly making up for all we had misunderstood, forgotten, or not attended in the previous four years.

For all this, our group of eight or so students bought him a tiny bottle of brandy, we were so broke, and admitted our ploy, to which his response was remarkably noble. One good practical teacher is worth scores of lectures and books.

Most of us learned all sorts of bizarre mnemonics to remember the causes of 'X' or the treatment of 'Y'. We were therefore good with lists, but abysmal with common sense On being asked a sensible question, to which a lay person could come out with an appropriate answer, we would start with the most obscure, and work from there. One eminent professor of surgery told us that, if asked in our finals what the signs of stomach cancer are, the first sign an examinee describes is Virchow's Node (a rare but usually diagnostic sign), that student would not only fail, but suffer actual physical violence!

An outstanding example one of my peers gave was his answer to the management of a hiatus hernia. This is the common herniation of the stomach up through the diaphragm causing, initially, symptoms of indigestion. His first reply was an Angelchik prosthesis, a fancy surgical technique very occasionally considered. The examiner retorted, 'What about a little antacid?'

Our patient examination techniques were little better. One way of testing a subject's co-ordination is to ask him or her to touch their nose with the index finger, then reach out to touch the doctor's index finger and back again, while the position of the doctor's finger is moved around. One of my friends misunderstood, and had the patient touching his own nose, and then the budding doctor's nose, instead of index finger, while he darted around varying the position of his head and getting poked in the eyes.

Life was not all work, however. As the studying became more intense, so did the partying. My housemates and I were invited to Hogmanay in the Scottish lowlands by one of the girls in our year, and journeyed up to her parents' huge farm over the border. One of our number celebrates his birthday on New Year's Day, though that year he didn't celebrate that day as he was unconscious. At around two in the morning he was seen to wax lyrical in an awful attempt at a Scots accent, 'On yonder hill I saw a cou, it must have moved it's not there nou,' then keeled over.

We carried him back to his bed, in a room which I had the misfortune to be sharing with him. After my drinking experiences after my A levels, I was slightly more sober than he, and I lay down on the floor beside the bed, as they were limited, to sleep. Minutes later I was roused by a foul nauseous smell, to open my eyes two inches from a pile of his vomit, as he had been careful not to soil the bed. This started a chain reaction, perhaps enhanced by the fear that I could have died from vomit aspiration, and not even my own vomit!

Most of the time we knew better, and a pint or two at the local pub after two or three hours revision each evening was the more normal way of relaxing. Time flew by, revision timetables were revised to become increasingly cramped, and in spring 1982 we started our final examinations; written papers first, followed by the clinical examinations. If one passed these, mainly with local examiners, a two or three month holiday followed. If not successful the first time, a month later those failed subjects would be retaken with external examiners. Failure then meant retaking in the autumn.

Fortunately, I was one of the 50 per cent or more who passed first time. Knowing your subjects was important, but equally important was *looking* as if you knew your subject: confidence.

The patients were wonderful. My main surgical case was a lady who had an aortic aneurysm leaking into the fourth part of the duodenum, presenting as an iron deficiency anaemia. This is exceedingly rare, but fortunately I asked her outright what was wrong with her, and she told me.

I was recommended to sit the honours paper in obstetrics and gynaecology, but as I had no other honours points collected, and therefore could not possibly be one of the 10 per cent or so who passed medicine with honours, I went to Ireland in my increasingly rickety car with Ewan and Danny instead.

During finals, many of my compatriots showed great resilience in the face of adversity. One fortunately gregarious girl, when discussing the oral contraceptive Pill with an eminent professor was asked, ‘Well, what kind of Pill are you on? You look like a bedworthy kind of girl!’

Even the few who were told to, ‘Come back, knowing rather more, to see me when the leaves are turning brown,’ bore their failure bravely. One of our year was told towards the end of his clinical exam that he had failed so far to impress his examiners, but would be given one last chance:

Question – ‘Imagine you are a GP, having seen a patient at his home with hypercalcaemia. The only phone is a call box, and you only have one 10 pence piece. You are requesting me to admit him. Tell me the symptoms you would describe.’

Answer: ‘Er ... erm ... er – pip, pip, pip!’

Result: ‘See you in November.’

For the majority who made it, the graduation day was a fine affair. In the evening we took over the Piccadilly Hotel in Manchester, and many of us invited our parents who, amazingly, had faith in us in the previous years, even when we did not.

A year book was given to each of us with photographs, and comments we were known for, documented inside. Apparently, my phrase for which I was known was, ‘To be on the safe side.’ I wasn’t sure if this accurately described me, and if so in what context…

My girlfriend for the previous two years or more was another graduate from my year. These pairings were not uncommon. Some couples even got married, and in a few instances they have even stayed married. My partner and I seemed fairly well suited in the medical school atmosphere, but we realised shortly afterwards that in the real world we were not, and we went our separate ways.

In that summer all seemed well. We could finally call ourselves doctors. I made some lifelong friends as, after all, we had in many ways grown up together in the previous five years. Although a few brave final year students had taken a week or two locum posts in that last year, not many of us really had much idea of what lay ahead. It was time to pay back some of the time and money that had been invested in us, and to actually start, at the age of 23, a real job.

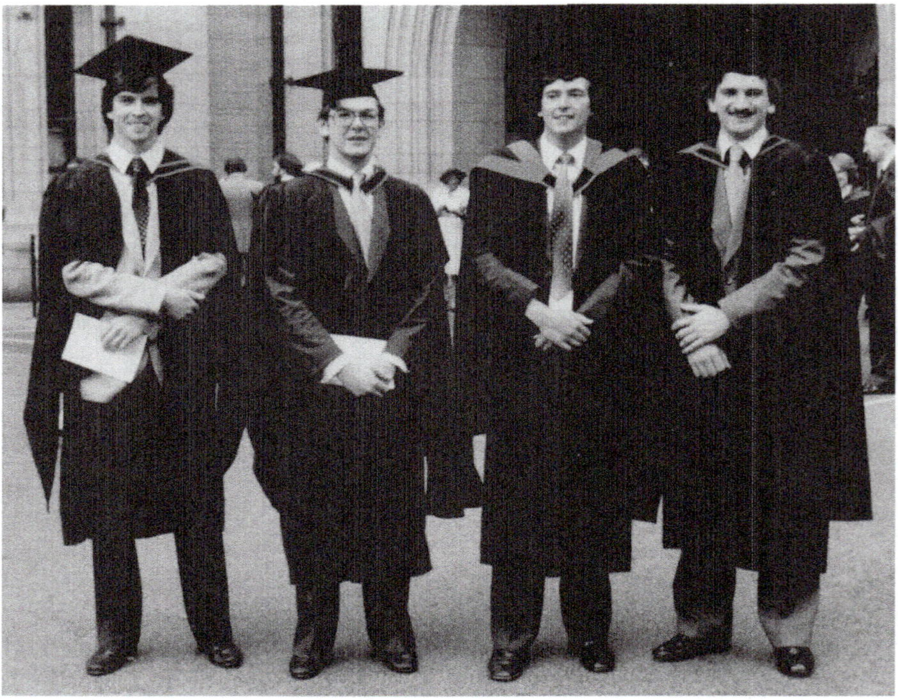

Danny, Ewan, Me, Graham, on our Graduation Day 1982

CHAPTER EIGHT

Halfway through the final year we were invited to apply for our pre-registration house officer posts. Although by passing our final exams we were qualified doctors at the end of the fifth year, one is required to spend six months in hospital medicine and six months in surgery, to find out what it is really like. Rather like passing one's driving test, the exams ensured one was relatively safe to start really learning to do what is required. Having no desire to climb the 10 to 15 year slippery career ladder in surgery, I applied for about four district general hospital surgical posts, which I thought I might enjoy, and might give me some useful experience for whichever branch of medicine I eventually landed in. In fact, one could usually guarantee more practical experience in such hospitals, rather than teaching hospitals. At the latter, although one got to work for some leading figures in their field, there were so many house officers, senior house officers, registrars, research registrars, and senior registrars, never mind consultants and professors, that practical experience was limited.

My first interview was in Preston, a place I had never previously visited, and I knew of only as an area where it rained when passing on the M6 motorway. However, the idea of three months' orthopaedics and trauma, of which there was plenty thanks to the road network, and three months' surgery, appealed to me. A large group of not-yet-qualified students sat nervously around a hideously carpeted postgraduate centre, designed to induce a migraine in anyone who hadn't already got a tension headache. No one spoke, even though some of us were from the same year in Manchester. Others came from Liverpool, Dundee, and elsewhere. Unable to bear the silence, one student, prominent by his height and, I learned later, by his personality, struck up a conversation with me. Later in the year, Brian and I were to find comfort in the fact that having secured similar posts, we were each as nervous of the job as each other, and everyone else.

Somewhat keener on general medicine, I applied for and obtained, for the following six months, a post in Hope Hospital, Salford, partly so as to give myself an opportunity to gain a few contacts for my no doubt brilliant medical future.

After what was chronologically a long holiday, which passed with what seemed like frightening speed, I drove on Sunday 1 August 1982 from Bramhall to Preston. Where the M61 joined the M6, a newly registered Ford Escort XR3 was concertinaed on the hard shoulder into about half its previous size. The awful truth that the next day I was going to have to deal with the occupants of such cars dawned on me, but I resisted the urge to vomit, and continued on to the newly constructed Royal Preston Hospital. The staff village was my home for the next six months, and I was pleasantly surprised. Those on rotas of a one in three, or worse, had free accommodation, small consolation though this was for unending working hours, I soon learned. (A 'one in three' meant working one evening and night in every three, and one weekend in every three from Saturday morning to Monday morning, as well as every weekday.)

From the switchboard office, I picked up my bleep, which is every doctor's ball and chain. In the coming years we learned to hate the high-pitched repetitive noises they issued as they disturbed meals, sleep, bowel movements, and every other conceivable bodily function. I collected my white coats and badge, and unpacked my stack of what I was soon to learn were practically useless text books. The next day, after no sleep at all, I walked out on to my first ward to realise that most of the regular nursing and medical staff knew we wouldn't have much idea, and would help us through those first days and weeks. Provided one did not pretend to know it all, and that one asked for help when needed, it was freely given. In fact, one's duties consisted mainly of clerking patients and organising investigations, while the senior house officer (SHO) decided an appropriate management of the trauma cases.

One or two of the less kindly disposed nurses had me doing what I was later informed were standard nursing duties, but this probably did me some good. In fact, some authorities feel that medical students should spend some time nursing, and others feel that we should spend some time as patients, which would probably be even more instructive.

I soon learned that trauma ranged from kids falling out of trees to elderly osteoporotic ladies breaking their hips. Unfortunately, whereas the children would be home the same or the next day, the elderly would occupy the same hospital bed for weeks or even months. It was upsetting to see someone's independence often disappear forever, first physically, and then mentally, as they became institutionalised, disorientated, and sometimes demented, in spite of their – and the hospital's – best efforts.

One poor soul who had been admitted with a fractured neck of femur, and who had lost all touch with reality, used to sit all day and night tapping the tray in front of her with her wedding-ringed finger shouting, 'Nurse please, nurse please,' for no fathomable reason. While she seemed to know little about this, the other patients on the ward and some of the staff were driven to their wits' end. The only variation was when someone encouraged her to shout, 'Clive please, Clive please,' instead, making it hard for me to concentrate on anything else. I understand she eventually got up, fell over, broke her other hip and died.

I enjoyed orthopaedics, partly due to the mainly straightforward approach of the doctors. There was little esoteric medical theory to get to grips with, which was refreshing after medical school. As one consultant physician since put it: 'Orthopaedic surgeons have the strength of an ox, and about the same IQ.' However, with my lack of skill in complicated matters practical, I could see this was not where I was destined, whereas I began to realise I enjoyed getting to know people, and their all-round medical situation. I tend to shy away from jargon, but I suppose this could be called holistic medicine.

I also enjoyed my three months in general surgery, even though this was a one in two rota. My consultants were both senior men, but were quite approachable. The patients were in awe of them. Though the consultants seemed quite awkward talking with the patients, they were completely at ease removing or reconstructing bits of them. They tried to communicate but it didn't always work. One patient, who was recuperating in his hospital bed, could see the college named after him out of his hospital window. He was remarking how pleasant that was, when the consultant followed with, 'Anyway, I hope it lasts longer than you do!'

The hospital social life was amazing. The seriousness of the work, and the hours of it, made most of us keen to make full use of our time off. This usually meant parties in one or other flat, consisting of large amounts of alcohol, music and, in the pre-AIDS era (just), promiscuity by a proportion of the residents. With the long working hours and short sleeping hours, both on and off duty, after a few months many of the junior doctors looked and felt like the living dead. Our consultants didn't seem to mind this, so long as we did the job well. In fact, they were very tolerant. At my first mess dinner I was trying to make polite conversation with one of our consultants when, during the soup course, a granary bun, complete with sesame seeds, flew over and bounced off his head. He simply grabbed his bun, and lobbed it in the direction of some of my contemporaries, from whence the original missile had come.

During my surgical post, I accepted admissions from the outside world, from GPs. On the whole they seemed a reasonable bunch who referred us appropriate clinical cases. I was not arrogant enough to think I knew what made up the often complex reasons for a patient's need for admission. The variety of people admitted, with their different presentations, made me think it might be even more challenging to try to come to a diagnosis in the community than it was in hospital, where we had the benefit of nurses, doctors, and a clean well-lit room to examine the patient. I also realised I enjoyed getting to know the patient as a person, more than focussing on one particular part of them. Surgery was satisfying, as a patient often came in quite unwell, had a procedure, and usually got better, but one never really got to know the owner of the offending appendix, breast lump, or gangrenous leg.

Even less appealing to me was the other speciality I was able to observe closely at that time – anaesthetics. This struck me as very dull, occasionally livened up with unexpected moments of crisis, where action taken within minutes decided whether someone lived or died. As one consultant in this field later put it to me, 'Ninety-five per cent of the time one wants to be somewhere else, and for the other five per cent of the time one wants to be anywhere else!'

Although having not even begun my six months of general medicine, I found myself drawn to general practice as a career choice. Hopefully, this was not due to the negative feelings I had for the lengthy training required for most hospital specialities. I was, however, beginning to realise that many of my colleagues a few years down the line were, at the age of thirty or more, still working one in two and one in three rotas, lacking sleep, becoming embittered by their lack of progress in their chosen branch of medicine, and distanced from their family and from reality by it all. The three years' security a structured GP training scheme would give me, and the fact that I liked Preston compared to many of the other hospitals I had encountered, led me to apply for a place on the vocational training scheme for general practice. This was to commence the following autumn, and was a widely respected scheme.

Four hospital posts of importance in a varied career ahead – general medicine, casualty, obstetrics and gynaecology, and paediatrics – all as a senior house officer were followed by a year as a trainee in general practice. At my interview I answered all the questions in as straightforward a way as I could, my only stumbling block being that I had quite honestly said I was a member of the British Athletics Club. I had joined as a means to get to know about forthcoming marathon runs, which were at the time popular among 'fun runners', though this now seems to be a contradiction in terms to me. I was asked how many international honours I had, and felt suitably inadequate.

There were sixty applicants for five places, a marked contrast from the situation at the time of writing this piece. Now there are sometimes fewer applicants than there are places, and some schemes have closed, due to the apparent unattractiveness a career in general practice currently presents. I was fortunate enough to be appointed, though some of the unsuccessful candidates then went on to make up their own schemes of equally and sometimes more interesting posts, interspersed with periods working or travelling abroad.

CHAPTER NINE

In February 1983 I temporarily left Preston to spend my six months pre-registration medical house officer's post at Hope Hospital in Salford. The genial old chap, an excellent clinician, whom I had been appointed to work for had been inconsiderate enough to retire, and had been replaced by a bright young man with a boyish enthusiasm for all things medical. The hospital smelled more of the mortuary, oddly placed near the entrance, than I had remembered, and the Victorian wards had seen better days. The only modern part of the hospital buildings were the twin nurses' and doctors' tower blocks, and my room had a radiator which clanged at night as the air pockets bubbled through it. Within weeks of arriving I so desperately needed a decent night's sleep following my on-call and socialising duties, I was reduced to audio-taping these nocturnal gurglings, to play back to the accommodations officer to convince her that a plumber was badly needed. They weren't too impressed, but when 56 continuous hours began from the next Saturday morning, one needed a decent night's sleep, particularly if the preceding week had seen at least one late night visit to a Manchester nightclub.

August and February are not good times to be admitted to hospital in England. This is when the junior doctors change posts, and get to grips with their new duties. In order to lessen the impact at Hope, the senior house officers changed after us, which in my case meant my immediate superior for the first fortnight was an experienced and no doubt academically bright, larger-than-life character, but whose inflated waistline matched his inflated opinion of himself. He took great pleasure in watching me flounder, then coming to the rescue.

I still remember the first medical patient I admitted. Armed with white coat, pockets full of little books like, *The House Officer's Survival Guide*, and a head crammed with useless facts, I marched down to casualty to see a large grey man, acutely short of breath, distressed and in pain, and sweating profusely. I then started sweating almost as profusely, as my SHO asked me to sort this poor chap out. Pulse weak, irregular, barely palpable, BP unrecordable, cold, clammy, and disorientated. I am, of course, referring to the patient here. I figured out he was in acute left ventricular failure, probably secondary to a myocardial infarction, confirmed by ECG. I was all set to start a number of blood tests and a chest X-ray when my senior smugly and correctly, of course, suggested treating the patient to ease his distress first. Intravenous analgesics and diuretics were given in fairly large doses, and miraculously the patient started to improve. This was very satisfying, and he went on to the score sheets to record Medical Team 1 : God 0 – so far. The scoreline often evened out, and some days we lost rather badly.

After two weeks my SHOs changed, and an immediately likeable character joined 'our team', who had a lovely way with patients, his medical colleagues, and particularly, it transpired, the nursing staff. Shortly to be taking the first part of his examination for membership of the Royal College of Physicians, he knew a huge number of facts, but also had an approachable helpful manner and an admirable calmness in all situations which, I quickly learned, was vital in effective management of critically ill patients. If the senior doctor on the spot, be it a cardiac arrest or an acute gastrointestinal bleed, is calm and clear in direction, others are too. Appearing flustered gets nobody anywhere.

In less immediately life-threatening situations he took himself and medicine in general less seriously. Instead of, 'On examination – overweight' or 'obese', he would think nothing of writing, 'mega abdomen' or 'mega mammaries'. On one occasion we admitted a middle-aged man with an unusual collection of neurological symptoms. My SHO conducted an extremely thorough examination, documented on five sides of A4 hospital paper, and including every neurological test I had heard of and quite a few I hadn't, and then he wrote, 'Diagnosis – either this chap has some very strange disease, or he is a loony!' Not the kind of thing one is encouraged to write in medical notes, though at the time I did become concerned regarding some of the other diagnoses and management decisions, not just at that hospital.

When an acutely ill elderly patient was admitted, after a full history and examination, and initial investigations, if the prognosis was poor, then 'NFR' was sometimes written in the notes: 'not for resuscitation.' This would mean that were the patient to deteriorate rapidly further, while all that could be done to ease any distress should be put into effect, overzealous measures such as calling the cardiac arrest team were not taken. I never remember feeling that an inappropriate decision was taken and it did mean that frail elderly folk could pass away with dignity rather than being jumped on by a resuscitation team, but I did feel that the patient and their families should have been more involved in the decision-making. I am sure this now is the case.

I always tried to discuss matters *with* the patient, rather than *over* them at the bedside or, worse, behind the curtain muttering away. I still hear reports from my patients in general practice, of groups of hospital doctors talking at them, then retiring to huddle in a small group occasionally nodding or shaking their heads, with only the odd word such as 'cancer' being audible to my patient.

At least with clear directives written in people's notes, for the medical and nursing staff to follow, patient management was decisive. There was nothing worse for the medical team, and particularly the nursing team who would be caring for the patient most of the time, to be unclear regarding a course of action, and I have always tried to make my patients, their families, and all the carers as informed as possible regarding a plan of action.

Although, after a few months, we were hardened to life-and-death situations, most of us would still treat our patients with respect and dignity. Comments regarding diagnoses, such as 'J.P.F.R.O.G.' ('Just Plain F***ing Run Out Of Gas'!) were rarely written in the notes, though occasionally spoken.

These months confirmed for me that I had taken the right decision in not following a career in general medicine. The teaching hospital world was not for me. I admire my colleagues who can elevate themselves to years of further examination and research, but the hierarchy I encountered did not appeal. I also felt that some of my senior colleagues had lost touch with reality.

There was a large ward where long-term patients would be transferred for further rehabilitation, often following major strokes. Sadly, many were never to become well enough again to be discharged from the hospital, never mind go home again. When the outlook was poor, or no signs of improvement had been forthcoming, a patient would gradually progress down the ward, as more recent admissions came in. There was a partition halfway down the ward, and once people had gone past this, they were informally and perhaps unkindly deemed by the staff to have then entered 'the departure lounge'.

These poor souls would sit by their bed all day, week after week, while nothing happened – except on Monday when I, and my fellow house officers, would get up at the crack of dawn to take blood tests on the off-chance a small variation in their bodies' biochemistry would be noted. This meant their tiny arms being turned black and blue as we desperately searched for a vein which wouldn't burst on contact with a needle, to have a test which, even if abnormal, would rarely alter the patient's management.

My consultant was fairly measured in his approach, but others were keen on what appeared to me at the time were minutiae. I recall one night admitting two men, not previously known to be diabetic, but who were very near death, both with blood glucose levels of 66mmol/1 (the normal being less than 10). After a 12-hour night of intensive observation and treatment from me, they survived, and by the morning they were almost conscious. My boss was away, and one of his colleagues was doing the ward round in his absence. I was so proud as I presented these two successes of mine, snatched from the jaws of death. He seemed almost off-hand, then asked me what their serum phosphate was, as this can vary in diabetic ketoacidosis. At that point I couldn't decide whether to tell him to shove his serum phosphate, or whether to cry, but instead I mumbled that I didn't know, as it wasn't immediately relevant and I was more concerned with saving their lives. These moments decided it for me. My career lay elsewhere.

We were all chronically tired as, again, it was a one in three rota, when, until spring arrived, we would often not go outside the hospital building in daylight hours for what seemed like an eternity. Occasionally, rumours of horror stories were heard around the doctors' mess, such as a tired doctor drawing up an antibiotic and mixing it accidentally with potassium chloride instead of water, and administering it to the patient who promptly had a cardiac arrest. Fortunately, the patient survived this dreadful experience. Nowadays, junior doctors work fewer hours, though when on call it must still be exhausting, and in order to reduce their hours they have to cover all sorts of different specialities at the same time.

Salford itself is not known for its affluence and, again, I could not help feeling a sense of injustice for many of the people I admitted who, through no fault of their own, were suffering deprivation so severe as to actually contribute significantly to their reasons for hospital admission. Many of them were non-complaining, and sadly resigned to their lot in life. The elderly gave up, the young at times turned to drugs and crime, and I felt that my efforts were small in comparison to their real needs.

I did venture occasionally back to leafy south Manchester, including one evening where I was the first ex-pupil to give the academic evening speech, and present O- and A-level certificates at my old school. This gave me time to reflect once more on the lucky start I'd had in life, compared to many of those living where I now worked.

Perhaps as a selfish antidote to my hospital experiences, I planned a holiday for my final two weeks of that period and for the following four weeks in between my pre-registration house officer's post finishing and the start of the GP training scheme.

CHAPTER TEN

Japan, I thought at the time, is about as near as I would ever get to seeing another world. Iain, my friend from junior-school days, had emigrated to play golf there professionally. This was a shrewd move. Although a scratch handicap golfer, I am sure he wouldn't mind me saying (wherever he is these days) he did not have that extra something needed to be outstanding in the professional competition world. However, being Western he was in great demand, as most things Western were. Even better, he was from the home of golf – Scotland.

As well as playing in tournaments, he gave golf lessons, and since one had to be staggeringly wealthy to play golf in Japan, he made friends with some influential people. At £100 for a round of golf, or £30,000 to buy membership of an average 18-hole golf course, people would pay large sums of money to improve their game. Iain became sponsored by a club manufacturer and, with his persuasiveness, would have people begging to spend £6,000 on a new set of their golf clubs if it would bring them even moderate success in their hobby, though for some it was more than that. Never, however, an obsession, as their work fulfilled that role. Intense, competitive and overwhelmingly energetic, the working population, predominantly men then, worked endless hours, from teeming out of the trains in the city in the morning, until they squeezed back in again some 12 or more hours later.

Having flown in via Alaska to Tokyo, I was greeted through the PA system at the airport to follow certain arrows – unless I had diarrhoea, in which case I was told to take another route. Fortunately my bowels were in good shape, so I uneventfully exited the airport into stifling humidity, where my old friend greeted me and took me in a mercifully air-conditioned car to his flat. This was, in fact, a tiny prefabricated box he was renting; the cost to buy would have been tens of thousands. The whole area he lived in reminded me of a scene from the film *Bladerunner.* All the wet, dark crowded scene needed was eerie electronic music, and Harrison Ford could have darted out of nowhere.

Being used to no sleep, we left shortly for the home of a Japanese family who had been kind to Iain and who had been good enough to invite us both over. I had been briefed this may happen, so having practised my chopsticks, and with a Royal Doulton china plate costing all of £20 as a gift, we arrived. They were impressed with the use of chopsticks, but absolutely bowled over by the china, and from that moment on couldn't be stopped from showering gifts in my direction. There was no Japanese for Clive Barker, so I was known as Kurieb Bowgao. I soon learned that the father of the family owned a large chunk of Yokohama, and that money literally was no object. We played golf, stayed in the Ryokan the emperor stayed in when on holiday, and all flew down to Hiroshima because I happened to mention that I felt I should go.

Less than 40 years since the atom bomb was dropped, I stood in what is now the Peace Park, trying to imagine the utter devastation of the bygone time. Having visited Germany less than 30 years after the end of the Second World War, and seen countless memorials all over the world, from little villages in rural England, to the Anzac memorial in Australia, I try not to forget how fortunate I am not to have had first-hand experience of the horrors of war.

On a lighter note, in a local restaurant not far from the Peace Park, something else I found moving, though in a different way, was the fish on my plate. Caught four minutes earlier from the sea, this poor creature flapped around on my plate after I had poked it with my chopsticks, thinking, not unreasonably, that it was dead. This, of course, caused great hilarity to the better-informed locals, though even when the head of the table leaned over and plucked the eye out, I smiled through clenched teeth and clenched pelvic floor muscles.

Apart from isolated occasions like this, I was made to feel most comfortable and the experience was a real antidote for the previous 12 months non-stop work. I put on a stone, became tanned, and must have become almost good-looking, as the amiable daughter of my Japanese family apparently became attracted to me. Heated debates in Japanese between my pal and the family surrounded me for the rest of the holiday, as he was quizzed as to the possibility of me staying in Japan. Though she was a lovely girl I had other plans in mind, and though her father would, I was told, buy me a hospital if I did stay, I felt I had to return. Anyway, I probably put her off with my awful singing in one of the karaoke bars, which had yet to journey to Europe. Frank Sinatra and the Bee Gees never sounded so bad, particularly after large amounts of whisky had been poured for me by overzealous hostesses at our private table.

So, tired, hung over, but enriched by the experience, I made my way back to England, and two years of hospital work which also left me tired, hung over, and at times enriched in other ways. For a brief moment I wish I had stayed, as on my jet-lagged return I found out my ex-girlfriend with whom I'd had a reunion prior to my departure to the Far East had forgotten me and, worse, our soft, daft but adorable spaniel had reached the end of her mortal coil. I also briefly thought my best mate was giving me the cold shoulder, as I phoned Preston to find out which part of my scheme I was to take up first and with whom, to be told by Ewan I was to be the Medical SHO for a dedicated, but dogmatic lady, who wanted things doing her way or else! My concern was met with monotone noncommittal comments down the telephone line.

'They have broken him,' I thought. 'He's been in the job one month and he has changed completely.'

What I didn't know was that he was, at that moment, in a room with his own consultant and it would not have been tactful to concur how frightening it might be working for one of his colleagues.

CHAPTER ELEVEN

Still, I was wrong if I thought a spirit could be broken in a month. It took about two weeks, or that is the way it seemed when on call for admissions. Twenty or more patients in a day, with coronaries, strokes, gastrointestinal bleeds, pneumonia – you name it, we took it. A production line of sick people all with their own concerns and needs which, apart from trying to keep them alive, I had little time to address. Their families would wait patiently, usually anyway, for word as to how they were doing, and often were dismissed with woefully inadequate explanations, as casualty was full of medical cases waiting to be assessed, and the sisters were breathing down my neck demanding to know when I was going to move my patients.

Even with a house officer and registrar on each team, we SHOs barely kept pace, and one's tone with reasonable requests for admissions from general practitioners became more and more exasperated. What was most frustrating was the lack of hospital beds to put these patients in, and an apparently even greater lack of concern from the administrators about this problem.

'Not my job – wouldn't know which patients could be moved,' would be the response to our desperate cries for assistance. I am afraid that from such experiences I developed a lack of respect for administrative and managerial staff which, in some cases, may well be unjustified, but receiving no help whatsoever when one hadn't slept for over 40 hours, and had a queue of acutely sick people needing beds, was extremely upsetting.

What I also found upsetting was my emerging lack of compassion. One almost felt relieved when a patient died, as this meant one less to look after, and a spare bed. Incredible perhaps to me now, but I don't know of a colleague in that job at that time who hadn't felt the same. One grew to hate the bleep, and on more than one occasion I found myself throwing it across my bedroom, having been woken after 10 minutes sleep. To keep awake I took to drinking large quantities of coffee, and smoking cigarettes, which I had done intermittently before, but this time I took it up seriously. I remember sitting in the doctor's office on a medical ward writing up the notes on a 40-year-old man who'd had a coronary. I felt I could be writing my own medical record for 15 years hence: lack of exercise, overwork, smoker.

On one occasion I chastised a patient having his third heart attack, that if he didn't stop smoking now he would be dead within a year. 'No threats,' I told him. 'Just fact.' I then pulled out my stethoscope from my white coat pocket, and out fell 20 Silk Cut King Size. On seeing him momentarily distracted from the pain he was in, I lied that they were confiscated from a previous patient.

I cringe now at my lack of respect for patients' dignity then, but we just didn't have the time. Every now and then, though, I would have a chastening experience, being humbled by one who had seen more life than I ever could. On storming down to casualty to see 'another stroke', I marched clinically in to see a little old lady in her eighties whose left side didn't work anymore. In my unnecessarily loud voice I asked her in the course of my history if she was married. She looked at me, almost forgivingly and said, 'No, I lost my fiancé in the war in 1917, and since then I never wanted none other.' I could only mumble that I was sorry, and vowed to treat people more sensitively – probably until I forgot to, shortly afterwards.

After my initial fears I did actually get on well with my consultant endocrinologist, partly because my predecessor had primed me with a 'Noddy's Guide to Diabetes', which I could refer to until I found my feet. My boss was also supportive of her junior staff, which helped considerably.

Life was not all work, though, and we did let off steam in a big way. Coach trips to a pub which had lock-ins until two in the morning, and served beer called Moonraker, were always well subscribed – until the pub got closed down, that is.

Ward nights out were popular too, but working on six medical wards and a coronary care unit meant that apart from the one in three nights and weekends on call, we were never in. On trying to figure out why I felt so awful around Christmas that year, I concluded that averaging four hours' sleep a night between work and socialising over a three week period was not good for one's health.

Ewan and I had a second floor flat, which constantly smelled like a pub, in one of the several identical residential blocks in the staff village. Apart from the standard water fights and irresponsible fire extinguisher lettings-off, one would also be able to play 'guess which room the shrieks of sexual ecstasy were coming from'. Not our flat, I hasten to say, nor did I encounter the girl with the pineapple rings, or the sex-to-music group.

My flatmate was unfortunate enough one night – or, more accurately, *drunk* enough – to wander into a flat thinking it was ours, only to enter what he thought was his bedroom to see sexual gymnastics being performed by a couple he had never seen before, and who, in turn, were wondering what he was doing in their flat!

On various nights out, even the more seemingly stern nursing and medical staff would let their hair down. One of my colleagues now describes a phrase which could sum up some of the more unexpected participants in off-duty revelries. One of the senior nursing sisters said to her, 'Just because I'm left on the shelf, it doesn't mean to say I haven't been taken down and dusted a few times!'

Certainly there was never a dull moment, though quite what all this had to do with a career in general medical practice I wasn't sure. We even used to pretend to be eccentric general practitioners phoning our mates on call, requesting to admit people with bizarre symptomatology, and managed to get each other quite irate. However, we would make sure this was only in a relatively quiet moment, in between inserting pacemakers, chest drains and performing lumbar punctures, and all sorts of other unpleasant investigations on other people.

CHAPTER TWELVE

Casualty was a thoroughly enjoyable six months, and comparatively civilised after my recent experiences. The working shift system meant that one was never on duty more than 12 hours at a time, an absolute luxury. The work was varied and, not being exhausted, one could really put one's heart into it: orthopaedics, medicine, surgery, and paediatrics.

All-round knowledge was required and if one felt out of one's depth there was a duty doctor in each of these specialities to refer to. Quite a lot of the presentations could have been dealt with in general practice, and the primary health care team got rather a bad name, and folk would turn up who 'couldn't get an appointment with their GP' requesting to be seen. I got quite a good idea of what life in general practice is like in that job, as one never knew what was going to present next – acute myocardial infarction, perforated duodenal ulcer, fractured tibia, febrile convulsion etc.

We also dealt with victims of their own and others' actions: drug abuse, overdoses, alcohol intoxication, assault, and self-inflicted injuries. One grew hardened to this sort of thing. Some poor souls in desperation would take to ingesting excessive amounts of medication to harm themselves. Others, to draw attention to themselves, would take minor overdoses, just to get themselves admitted to hospital, and to generate some sympathy from their boyfriend/girlfriend/parents, or anyone. Unfortunately, what they didn't realise was that even small amounts of drugs such as paracetamol could be lethal. It is well documented that 12 to 20 of such tablets taken at once can kill, and have done so to adolescents only wanting to worry their partners or their parents.

While that was upsetting, I found myself increasingly annoyed and unsympathetic with characters, usually adults, who would repeatedly 'overdose', and then demand to be admitted to hospital, so distracting the medical and nursing staff from those patients who through no fault of their own needed urgent care. One man during my shift was admitted with his thirtieth paracetamol overdose. We thought of making him an anniversary cake made of Parvolex, used to treat such cases.

Sometimes, when busy with genuine casualties, I would dearly liked to have turned him away but, of course, we could not. On Friday and Saturday nights I could count the sober patients I saw on the fingers of one hand. I became disgusted with the people who would brawl in the street, on the way to hospital, and in the casualty waiting room, then expect to be patched up so they could do the same the following weekend. Of course, there were many victims of uninvited aggression, and I came to abhor even more vehemently the mindless vandalism inflicted on innocent parties who happened to be in the wrong place at the wrong time. We also saw many victims of domestic violence, usually women and children.

Eighteen months after my nauseous worrying, seeing a road traffic accident on the motorway on the way to start work, I was now the first point of hospital contact for the victims of these crashes. The ambulance crews were so efficient, my patients were usually stabilised in splints and collars with airways open and oxygen masks applied. I could relatively coolly assess the situation and take bloods, organise X-rays and set up intravenous infusions, as well as contact relevant specialities quickly. Twelve years later, of course, with the extension of paramedic skills, intravenous infusions are already set up and appropriate drugs given, so that patients have had a large proportion of their treatment before they ever reach hospital.

If patients reached hospital alive then their chances were reasonable, though a significant proportion didn't. Certifying people 'dead on arrival', particularly children, was desperate. I recall seeing a little boy who had been run over by a motor vehicle. He was already obviously dead, but I insisted the staff emergency-bleeped the paediatrician as I couldn't comprehend this little life was extinguished. Now my own children must be tired of my road safety lectures, but I make no apologies for that.

Before the days when emergency ambulances were common and paramedics were highly trained, we had an emergency ambulance called 'India One'. This was a rickety predecessor of today's intensive treatment units on wheels. The ambulance was many years old by the time I came to staff it.

Hence the suspension was going, and the fancy helmets with 'Doctor' and 'Nurse' written on them were not worn but used to vomit into going over bumps and around sharp bends. By the time we reached our destination we usually needed resuscitating even more than the patient.

One of my colleagues arrived at a scene, with his last meal surprisingly still in his stomach, to see a collapsed patient and leapt heroically out of the vehicle armed with the defibrillator, to see an obviously dead pedestrian lying on the pavement. Surrounded by anxious onlookers he felt he had to do something, so attempted to shock the patient back to life, only to find that the defibrillator didn't work. I even heard tell of the ambulance being fitted out in one of the hospital garages, being adorned with a big blue flashing light on top. On its first emergency call it left the garage, and left the light behind as it was swept off the top of the roof, as the doors were not high enough. Not too impressive!

During this time I had cause to be grateful for other people's life-saving skills, as on Easter Sunday 1984 I very nearly died. Three friends and I decided to go away for Easter Saturday and Sunday, to Bala in North Wales. Danny and Graham and Pete and I took two windsurfers, and we set off in high spirits to arrive early in that village for a fry-up in one of the local cafés. The eerie lady serving our cholesterol on a plate warned us about the hazards of Lake Bala.

'You want to be careful there,' she said, 'deepest lake in Wales, very cold at this time of year. People drown in there, you know.' She went on to tell us of every tragedy in recent years in the vicinity, which of course we shrugged off and bade her farewell and headed towards the lakeside.

Saturday was a lovely sunny day and I found my overconfidence quickly, wearing my mate's wetsuit and lifejacket. Three of us stayed over while Graham headed back as he was working in Wrexham that Sunday night in casualty. The Sunday started quite nicely, and after an outdoor weekend away from our respective hospital jobs, we thought about packing up. Impulsively, I wanted one last go, and hopped on to the windsurfer for a final foray along the lake shore. Within minutes the sun went in, the wind blew cold, and blew me straight out into the middle of the lake, where I was becalmed.

No lifejacket. Why hadn't I remembered to put it on? Still, I could get myself back. Wind blew harder. Too proud to shout for assistance. Up on to the board, blown off again. Now my friends were out of earshot anyway. Try to swim pulling the board – too heavy. Back on to the board. Fell in again.

Shoulder clicked. Getting very cold. Started shouting for help. No one heard. Tried to windsurf back once more. On to the board, held sail, fell backwards hitting the board as I went in. Left shoulder dislocated. The time elapsed between landing in the freezing water with my shoulder out of joint, and reaching up to the board with both arms, and lifting myself on to it must have been barely more than three seconds, but if I had taken any longer I am sure I would have been part of the flora and fauna at the bottom of Lake Bala. It may sound overdramatic, but this is exactly how it happened. I clung to the board literally for dear life. I was seizing up, and if I had gone in again that would have been it. The wind was causing the water to lap around the board tipping it repeatedly. Apart from the wind and the water, there was total silence.

It's strange what one thinks about when death seems imminent. I remember clearly thinking that although I'd had a good life, I hadn't left much behind me, not much evidence of my existence and, with a desperate will to live, I started shouting like crazy. Barely distinguishable above the waterline, Danny and Pete began to realise that all was not well. They sent out a would-be hero in a tiny inflatable dinghy. Paddling frantically, he made slow but steady progress towards me. Fortunately he didn't get there quickly enough, as I think I would have pulled us both in. In the meantime, what seemed like the only other craft on that huge lake sailed quite close, shouting to ask if I was all right. I replied weakly that I was not – most certainly not. A father and son in a catamaran drew skilfully alongside my now rigid torso lying flat on the board, and instructed me to climb aboard.

'But I can't move,' I retorted, and I couldn't. Over an hour in these conditions, and a now useless left arm meant I was helpless. 'Please don't let me go in,' I begged. They drew me gently alongside, and tried to haul me on to their craft. I went in the water. I stuck out my right arm. They grabbed it and hauled me, with no help from myself, on to the catamaran. Forgetting the windsurfer, we sped to the shore as I curled up in a small ball on the plastic sheet between the hulls of their boat. I staggered on to the shore, and into Pete's car, and we headed off to Wrexham casualty, where Graham was soon to come on duty. I didn't care how much it hurt now. I was on dry land.

In the casualty department I tried stoically to sit in the waiting room, but must have looked pretty awful, as the sister made me come immediately through into the treatment area. There I was given Entonox (nitrous oxide), and the orthopaedic registrar relocated my shoulder. Glad to be alive, and high on the gas, I think I nearly kissed him. Fortunately, at this stage, they didn't know I was a casualty officer myself.

I tried to contact the people who saved my life that day, but I had only got the scantiest of details from them in my distress, and never did get to thank them personally.

Back at my own place of work I kept my arm in a sling for a week or two. I had given up resting it in a body bandage and sling for weeks on end after the first time that didn't work at medical school. However, lifting myself on to that board, necessary though it was at the time, had damaged my whole shoulder permanently, so I thought I should rest it for a while. I could not therefore wear a white coat effectively, so when I called in patients over the PA system in casualty, they walked straight past me thinking I was another patient. To restore their confidence took some doing. I patched up children who had fallen out of trees in the spring and summer, and their parents who had DIY'd holes into themselves, or lopped bits of fingers off on corned beef tins.

In the quieter moments we used to keep ourselves and others amused by planting patient cards with absurd names for our colleagues to call out over the PA system. Looking back, I am surprised how gullible we were, but in the routine of work one wasn't always as astute as could have been hoped. Hence, Annette Curtain, Teresa Green, and Hugh Janus were instructed to proceed from the waiting room, where the unsuspecting casualty SHO would be wondering why no one was answering their call. It all seems rather juvenile now, but it lightened up the more serious moments.

The hospital social life continued apace, but it began to dawn on me that in a little over a year I would be entering general practice, and I wouldn't know anyone other than the doctors and nurses in the hospital environment. Although happy in my life in my mid twenties, working and partying, I do remember thinking that there must be more to life than this. I lived in an unreal environment, surrounded by other young people, mainly women, which gave a rather skewed angle of one's observations of life.

My erstwhile windsurfing colleagues and I went on a gloriously sunny two-week Greek island-hopping adventure that summer. I was concerned to discover that my not-so-amazing personality, which made me comfortable in the hospital environment where I knew and worked with most people there, was very mundane to total strangers. Feeling relaxed and inebriated, I would try to wax lyrical when seeking to impress members of the opposite sex. On balmy starry Mediterranean nights, I would stare up at the sky and explain how insignificant I felt against this vast universe. I would continue, 'To think that the light we are seeing from most of those distant stars set off from its source before we were even born, and since then it has been travelling at 186,000 miles every second.'

The people I was trying to impress must have also thought I was insignificant, as by the time I had finished marvelling, they had usually gone home! The only time I did manage to attract an inquisitive look was from a girl I was trying to chat up above the blaring noise in Scorpion's Disco in Ios. I couldn't help noticing her gaze drifting downwards, but unfortunately this was only because she had noticed, unlike me, that there was a large gash in my trousers and also my left thigh, from where blood was oozing. I had fallen in the dimly lit street, and was so keen not to injure my shoulder, I had forgotten to protect the rest of me.

On a previous holiday some months before, Ewan and Dermot and I had spent a week in Tenerife, where we experienced the worst weather they'd had there for six years. Fortunately, on that occasion, and because my two friends had girlfriends back home, we knew better than to try to impress. Instead, we found a local bar at which we spent most of the holiday, looking like slightly younger versions of the three characters from *Last of the Summer Wine*. In spite of keeping ourselves to ourselves, we still managed to look rather pathetic when we decided to have a sauna and massage, which the hotel, mainly populated by Germans, offered. Although such facilities can in some places have dubious connotations, this was of course completely innocent, in spite of some of our friends' suggestions to the contrary since.

Trying to look as if this was something we regularly did at home, we went for a sauna and drew lots as to who went first for the massage. I think I won, and therefore chose to go last. This was a bad move, as by the time for my massage came, I had been in the sauna an hour and a half!

Clinically dehydrated, I staggered into the room for my massage, where I was horrified to be told to remove my swimming trunks by the masseuse. In return, she gave me a towel the size of a small ladies' handkerchief which, after all that time in the sauna, was easily enough to hide my modesty. Unfortunately Ewan, having gone first, had opted for oil as the massage medium, which dried up after about 10 of the 30 minutes. This meant that virtually all of one's body hair was depilated, and any soothing effect of the massage was completely lost.

On returning to Preston, after our Greek holiday, I decided to join the local tennis club. I couldn't play very well, but at least it was a way of meeting people outside medicine and nursing. On Saturday 30 June 1984 I got quickly knocked out of the Captain's Day competition, but plucked up the courage to go to the dance in the evening. There I met one of the senior nurses who had looked after me as I found my feet in casualty. We got chatting, and Barbara introduced me to the girl with whom I was to spend the rest of my life.

Her daughter Carole had been absolutely certain she would have nothing to do with doctors outside hospital life, but unfortunately for her I was hooked, from that moment. We chatted for a short while and I found out she was a sister on the special care baby unit in Sharoe Green Hospital, where I would soon be working. Although she was very pretty, I found myself attracted by something else. We just seemed to talk so easily, and everything around me seemed to fade into the background and only she was in focus. Perhaps this was due to the alcohol I had consumed, but I doubt it.

CHAPTER THIRTEEN

Soon enough I had finished my casualty stint, and I moved hospitals to start six months' obstetrics and gynaecology. I vividly remember walking on to the labour ward at the beginning of the first day of this experience. Although these environments are now referred to as 'delivery suites', I think the former title more accurately describes them.

After introducing myself to the midwives as they bustled by, I was directed towards the appropriate rooms where there were three ladies waiting to have labour induced by breaking their waters.

'Well,' I explained, 'if any of them have a sprained ankle, I'm your man.' This was the problem with the scheme of rotating around posts. One would become proficient at one job after six months' experience, only to move to another about which one hadn't a clue. I felt even more sorry for the patients, nurses, and middle grade doctors, who had to patiently put up with our ineptitude. It was over three years since I had performed any practical obstetrics, and then only minimally. Now I was the one to whom patients', partners', and midwives' concerns were addressed.

At first, this basically consisted of being a messenger for those concerns to be passed on to my senior medical colleagues, but as with most things I slowly but surely got to grips with the situations. Having said that, in this job everything was so slimy and messy, in particular the babes, they were literally difficult to get to grips with. I never actually dropped a baby but one always had that fear! My feet used to get fairly wet too, as I found out on that first morning when inducing labour by rupturing the membranes. The liquor gushes out in a waterfall, to find a one inch gap between the bottom of the protective gown and the top of your wellingtons. Apart from these unscheduled footbaths, I thoroughly enjoyed my experiences, probably as most of us never cease to marvel at how wonderful it is seeing babies born.

For the women giving birth, 'wonderful' is not usually the expression they used to describe the experience. I occasionally found my enthusiasm dulled, usually at four o'clock in the morning, as I shuffled towards the maternity block from my quarters, to hear the freezing night air pierced by shrill cries of, 'Get the f***ing thing out, I can't take any more!'

The biggest problem were the fathers-to-be. Often women were accompanied by their mothers, sisters, or female friends who seemed to have a kind of empathy with the young mother-to-be. Many times they were helped by their boyfriend or husband, who were usually reasonably sensitive to their loved one's needs. Sometimes, however, they were interfered with by boorish males who had no idea what was going on, but were more concerned about how the experience was for *them*, rather than the mother or the baby.

I almost had to restrain myself from, for the first time in my life, hitting a man whose wife was going through hell in the middle of the first stage of labour. This was because when I gently suggested to the lady that a little pain relief might ease her discomfort and help her baby's progress, he butted in saying, 'My wife and I don't believe in pain relief, do we dear?' Had she not been so incapacitated I think she would have hit him herself. Another man, on guidance being given by the midwives regarding how he could best help and be involved, retorted, 'I'm not used to taking orders' – having previously been in the Armed Forces. Why these people couldn't just do the decent thing and faint like in the old days I couldn't understand. I also became impatient with the men who quipped, 'Couldn't just sew her up a bit tighter, could you doc?' while I repaired the vaginal tears or episiotomies. This was a major part of the job. Thankfully, most midwives suture when necessary nowadays, but not then. And I actually became quite proficient, even for those ladies who had understandably tried to avoid having an episiotomy, only to tear horribly at the last minute. I spent Christmas morning crouched at one lady's bottom end singing carols while I worked. Fortunately, she was high on Entonox and I was high on sleep deprivation.

On more than one occasion in the following months, I was stopped in the street by women whose faces I didn't recognise, but who informed me that I had assisted their little one into the world and repaired everything afterwards.

On Boxing Day that year I got to admire first-hand the response time of the Fire Service to a fire alarm on the labour ward. I had been chatting to Ewan on the phone, and subconsciously started fidgeting with a screw on what had not registered as the fire alarm. Out popped the glass and off went the alarm. I remember wondering where the incident may be occurring, until minutes later in rushed several firemen, in masks and carrying oxygen equipment. With a sheepish grin, and hoping that I wasn't going to be charged several thousand pounds for the call-out, I apologised as profusely as I could.

I enjoyed getting to know most of the mums and some of the dads, though on less happy occasions it could be deeply upsetting. Most people reasonably expect a healthy, happy baby and mum at the end of the day, and usually this is the result, not due to any medical or nursing heroics, but due to nature. However, sometimes tragedies happen and when they do it is devastating. One day mum and babe can be progressing well, and the next day or even hour both can be in danger. Although modern obstetrics, midwifery, and paediatric practice have improved the outlook greatly compared with decades ago, they cannot always guarantee all will be well. There is no easy way to tell someone their baby has died, and even now I can only guess what it is like to lose a little one whose life has barely started.

Although we never lost a mum during my stay, one or two came fairly close. Haemorrhage during and immediately after birth can be torrential but, like in previous jobs, by keeping calm and thinking straight the correct measures will usually rectify the situation. I do remember seeing one lady have a fit, due to greatly elevated blood pressure, for which the immediate treatment was intravenous Valium. Though outwardly in control, I couldn't help wishing I could have some of the Valium first!

In fact, the job had a few scary moments, not least of which was because we were based on two sites. Our gynaecology patients were a mile or two down the road, so when my senior colleague had to go there I was the only doctor on the maternity unit. Towards the end of the job I felt more comfortable about this, but on one occasion when the senior members of my team were occupied with an emergency at the other hospital, a lady with a breech presentation baby was delivering. These were not that common and my experience was limited. Sitting in the sister's office revising from a text book how I was supposed to deliver this baby was not a comfortable feeling. No wonder I wore brown trousers for most of that six months.

Fortunately, mainly due to the midwives' skill again, all was well. I also got an inkling at that testing time of what paediatrics had in store, as this was set on three sites, so sometimes there was no paediatrician at difficult or complicated deliveries, so I had to double up. Even tiny newborns are often fighters and survivors, so heroics weren't often needed, but the first few times I intubated a baby to assist breathing, the adrenaline was certainly flowing. In fact, one of my colleagues described his 'Law of neonatal resuscitation'. The babe's heart rate plus the paediatrician's heart rate always equals 200. That is, a normal neonatal heart rate of 140 was accompanied by a steady SHO's heart rate of 60 beats per minute, but when a babe showed distress or collapsed with an abnormally low heart rate the doctor's went up and up!

This wasn't helped by the heat on the resuscitation equipment to keep the tiny patient warm, and sweat would pour down, to pool in your wellies along with the stale liquor. Added to this, the task of getting meconium out of a baby's mouth and lungs (if it had opened its bowels just before being delivered), could make the whole thing a pretty nauseating experience.

I think this is what put me off home deliveries. Apart from the fact that unforeseen problems can arise, the whole procedure is just plain messy. The parents' bed is never the same. We did take mums who had tried for home deliveries but had got too tired or had complications and who had to come into hospital. I tried to be as sensitive as I could as it was a big disappointment for them, but most felt that so long as the baby was all right it was for the best. Since then I have taken part in a few home deliveries, and many at the local GP maternity unit.

The best experience of all at this time was getting to know Carole. I recognised her as soon as I started the job, and as the special care baby unit (SCBU) was in the maternity block I let no opportunity go astray. I dreamed up all sorts of excuses to get to see her, the first being to watch a lumbar puncture being performed by my paediatric colleagues. I hoped she would think I was particularly conscientious, as my own job in the obstetrics department was busy enough. I 'accidentally' bumped into her at the canteen and several other places in the hospital. My persistence paid off, and within a respectable amount of time – two weeks, which seemed like a year – we went out together, though not as a date as such.

I called around anxiously at her parents' house where she lived, and her father Bert answered the door. Before I could get a word in edgeways, and as she had omitted to tell him I was calling, he thought I had come for the tennis club keys, which they looked after. I blurted out that I had, in fact, come for his daughter. In spite of this surprise, I was lucky enough to be accepted with warmth and friendship beyond that which any budding son-in-law could usually expect. Come to think of it, most of Preston at some time or other seems to have been welcomed into the Turner household over the years.

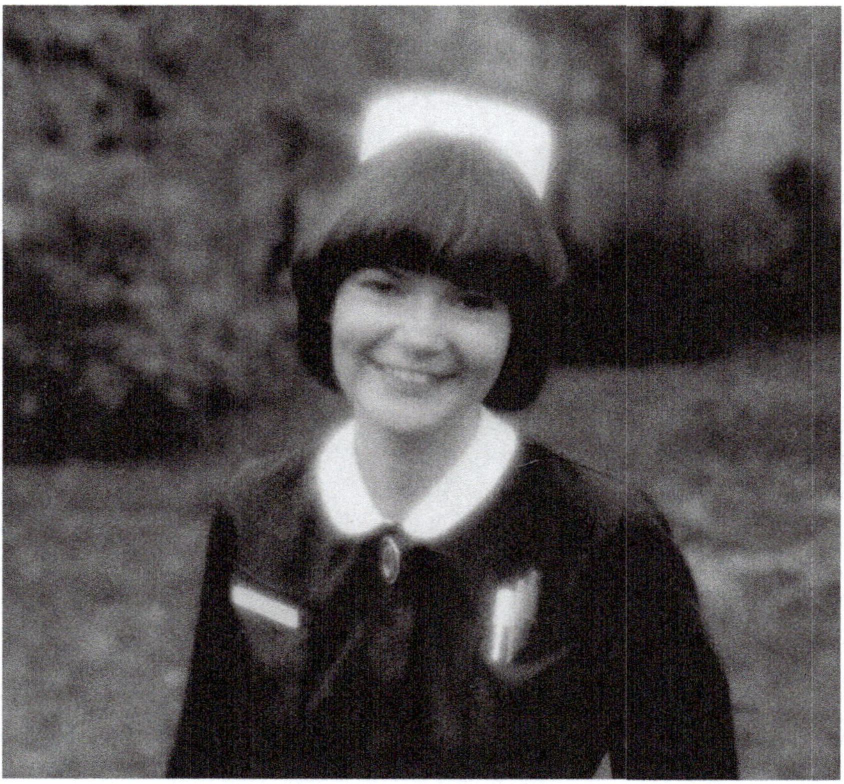

Carole (1984) shortly after we met

At that time I was living in the hospital quarters, in a room which had central heating pipes, seemingly for the whole hospital, going through it. Although they didn't make a noise this time, there were only two settings:

boiling hot and off. Even with all the windows open it was too hot when on, but was freezing when off. A happy medium was all windows open, and blankets lagging the pipes. After our first evening together I asked Carole back to see my lagging, but of course she declined.

Only due to my persistence, and my assurance of honourable intentions, did she eventually accept, and was of course fully justified in her trust. From then on we really hit it off. She did waver once, on that first evening, when I told her that I had a confession to make. This was that I occasionally still smoked a cigarette, though she feared that I was going to say I was, in fact, married! What little spare time we had at work, we seized the opportunity to see each other. We were the Mills and Boon characters of the hospital: 'Their eyes met across an incubator in which a tiny vulnerable babe lay sleeping.' We were teased mercilessly, but I don't think either of us minded. Once I started my paediatrics attachment we were, of course, working together.

CHAPTER FOURTEEN

The thought of the minuscule babes I was to be responsible for made me lie in my morning bath longer than usual the first day of my paediatrics post. 'Perhaps if I stay here long enough and just don't go in, no one will notice,' I thought. But as the water went cold, and the foam bubbles burst along with the confidence I had built up in obstetrics and gynaecology, I knew I could postpone it no longer. Another new job – another new experience.

After a slightly faltering start, I found my feet, and those feet were soon to be pounding faster than I had anticipated. My twenty-sixth birthday, on call, one week into the job. First stop, Preston Royal Infirmary – to be present at any planned caesareans and carry out any necessary tasks on SCBU. Next stop, Sharoe Green Hospital to do the same. Unfortunately, on my way to a caesarean section for twins my Vauxhall (again) Chevette conked out – total loss of power. I ground to a halt outside someone's drive, nearly a mile to the operating theatre I was supposed to be in. I leapt out of the car cursing wildly and, waving my stethoscope in the air, flagged down a passing car.

'Get me to Sharoe Green Hospital, I'm a doctor!' I shouted in my most dramatic fashion. Amazed, the lady driver let me in and took me straight there. I charged into the operating theatre to be mightily relieved to see two strapping newborn twins, perfectly healthy, and in fact in a better state than I was. After a quick rest I ran back to my car, only to find a calling card secured beneath the windscreen wiper. 'The Reverend has called and leaves his regards,' said the vicar's calling card. The type was crossed through, however, and written in ink over this were the words: 'Do you mind if I park in my drive?'

Provided I hadn't had major transport problems, I found myself quite competent at helping the small arrivals get to grips with extra-uterine life. Usually, problems could be predicted so I was around in good time to await the delivery of often surprisingly hale and hearty screaming infants.

Sometimes, though, white or grey babes would arrive floppily into the world, when all eyes turned to yours truly. Not breathing, low heart rate – do something! Initially, I was so keen to do something that I was correctly reminded by one father to at least let the mum see her baby, as I whisked it off to the resuscitaire. Start clock. Minutes count. In fact, seconds count. I was only too aware that once anything over two to three minutes had passed, the little mite I was trying to help might suffer for the rest of its life if I didn't get an adequate oxygen supply going, via a mask or an endotracheal tube. The father, midwives, and obstetricians would gather round to watch what was going on.

Usually the outcome was favourable, and a little croaky cry was greeted with relief and smiles all round (none more than mine). Very occasionally, though, no matter what one did the babe's heart rate would not come up, but slow further and eventually stop. After half an hour or more of doing everything one could think of and calling one's senior colleagues to help, we would have to stop our efforts.

Seeing a lifeless little baby spreadeagled on all this high-tech equipment which had made no difference at all, and stopping the clock and turning off the oxygen supply made us feel so inadequate. I still can't find the words to describe the feeling of wrapping up the still bundle in a blanket to take to its mum and dad.

It sounds selfish to describe one's feelings at times like this, when I can only guess what the families were going through. We doctors and nurses could gain some comfort in stressful times from the fact that we could all support each other.

As most babes did well, and because most children in general are made of strong stuff, paediatrics was generally a happy experience. I got on well with the patients, perhaps because my mental age was nearer theirs, and I enjoyed relating to their families. The infants and children who were admitted on to our third site, the Royal Preston Hospital, were a pleasure to see, and because they usually got better by themselves, were an antidote to the more serious cases we would see. Even these were rewarding to treat as we could usually do something for them.

My first admission in paediatrics was a child who'd had a non-resolving chest infection for two weeks, and who had given a large cough on the morning of admission, and suddenly gone acutely breathless and blue. I was very pleased with myself to elicit that he had lost a biro top a fortnight earlier while sucking on it. It had lodged in a lower lobe bronchus for two weeks, and then been dislodged by his cough to completely obstruct the whole of his lung on the other side, meaning that when I saw him he was functioning on half a lung. The offending object was removed with considerable skill by a bronchoscopist and an anaesthetist, and then we both made a total recovery.

During this period I also became a strong believer in the vaccination programme in this country. I have still never personally seen any evidence of lasting problems from immunisations, but I saw a couple of little ones with irreparable lung and brain damage due to the awful effects of the illness which is whooping cough.

Since then, other conditions have become less common due to these programmes. One such is epiglottitis. This is an infection causing swelling of the fold of tissue at the entrance to the trachea, usually caused by a bacteria, Haemophilus B. This is now protected against by the Hib vaccine, which also protects against this kind of meningitis. I have only seen one case of epiglottitis, and I never want to see another.

I was on call on Easter weekend 1985, having had three hours' sleep on the Friday night and three on the Saturday night, and I was praying for a rest by late evening on Sunday. Just as I was about to tuck into my takeaway tea, my bleep sounded. The casualty SHO had a little boy who looked ill, but she couldn't pinpoint why. I trudged down to the casualty cubicle to see a deathly white child cradled in the arms of his father, a vicar who had been giving the evening sermon when his boy had become ill. The youngster was making an ominous croaking sound, and looked dreadful. My tiredness dissipated and I rang my registrar and the anaesthetist on call. It is well documented that interference can precipitate complete obstruction of the airway, and then the only answer is an emergency tracheostomy – not easy in a small child.

Sure enough, the diagnosis was epiglottitis, and our little patient was transferred to the intensive care unit where we carefully set up a drip and intravenous access for antibiotics. After a sleepless night for us all, he slowly came back from the brink. By Easter Monday morning, when I handed over to my colleague on call that day. having had six hours' broken sleep in the last seventy-two, I felt satisfied that I had experienced the highs and lows of hospital medicine, and that I'd had enough of chronic sleep deprivation.

Of all my jobs over the preceding three years, I most enjoyed paediatrics, and if I hadn't chosen the path of general medical practice, I might have given it a go. The consultants were very approachable and supportive, the children were lovely, and the involvement of those in the child's environment gave me an opportunity to explore the varying mechanics contributing to a medical situation. Usually this was positive though, of course, physical and sexual abuse were being increasingly recognised, and drug abuse was beginning to rear its ugly head. I found myself feeling confident and in control, and towards the end of the six months I recall conducting the ward round with a nurse, also a good friend, neither of us older than 26 years, with Live Aid in the background, when we both suddenly realised that we were responsible for the well-being of all these patients. While trying to be serious we cracked up laughing, but we soon composed ourselves as we realised we really could do it. A very satisfying feeling.

Carole and I became closer and working together was a pleasure. She had the art of suggesting certain aspects of management, guiding me in the right direction and yet still making me feel as if I was involved in the decision-making process. This has continued in our married life together. In addition, then and now, I seem to have the energy and impetuous nature to come up with all sorts of plans and schemes, and Carole will filter out what is appropriate and what is not. She is the calm around which I rapidly orbit.

I knew that I had met someone very special, and although impulsive in less important matters, I appeared to be of a more cautious nature when it came to really major decisions. I didn't feel ready to commit myself forever, even though I knew I was in love. I explained to her that I had the impression that our friends and families thought we would soon become engaged, as we were so obviously right for each other. This, I felt, put me under some pressure. In fact, the only pressure was from myself.

Carole, of course, was perfectly satisfied to take life's events at whatever pace they occurred and enjoy them, rather than agonising about what one should or should not do, as I did in those days. How I could be conceited enough to think that she would want to spend the future with such an indecisive self-centred man I am still not sure. I was brought quickly back down to earth by the speed with which Carole got on with her life and bought a flat into which she settled so fast it almost made my head spin. I moved into my unfurnished rented housing association flat for my GP trainee year. I remember standing solitarily in it, suddenly realising independence wasn't that great after all!

CHAPTER FIFTEEN

Early on in the hospital component of my vocational training scheme, I had organised my year as a GP trainee (now referred to as registrar) with a five-doctor practice in Bamber Bridge, on the A6 between Preston and Chorley. The senior partners were a married couple who lived in the house to which the practice building was adjoined. The practice had been founded by the senior man's father many years before, who practised, I understand, well into his seventies until his eyesight failed. His son carried on the family tradition and he was well in his sixties when I joined, and he would have continued into his seventies had compulsory retirement at 70 not been introduced.

His wife was a trainer in general practice, and one of the lads in my year became her trainee. She was a very strong character, as no doubt one had to be in the days when women doctors were not that common. She also battled for years against facial cancer, undergoing extensive surgery, and recently succumbed shortly after retirement.

My prospective trainer was a gentle approachable chap in his early forties who, shortly after my appointment, died suddenly of a heart attack. The next most senior partner stepped in, and went to the trouble of gaining recognition as a trainer. Dave is a sound character with both feet planted firmly on the ground. Liked by his patients for his straightforwardness and honesty, he was a good role model for me.

The Royal College of General Practitioners has achieved a great deal for doctors and their patients but, as with many similar bodies, sometimes it is seen as removed from the reality of everyday general practice. Dave was not a member of the College – it was unusual, therefore, for him to be approved as a trainer – and he had a healthy scepticism of academia and 'holier than thou' approaches. The other two partners were little older than me, and offered me a great deal of help.

The premises were bare and cramped, but the atmosphere informal. The senior partner's dog would roam around the waiting room and often into the surgeries when consulting. The doors were not very effectively sound-proofed, a problem for my patients and me, as my voice is notoriously loud. In fact, since then my current partners have said they have picked up a few interesting phrases from my surgery, and one even says that when in the room next to me, he could just open and close his mouth and appear to be spouting words in consultation. Fortunately, since then, we have moved into more soundly proofed premises.

As a trainee, sitting in a consulting room observing general medical practice is, after a day or two, not very stimulating, and to any budding GP I would say do not judge by this experience. For a start it is a false situation, because of the very fact that an observer is there; most patients change their demeanour, and to a degree the doctors change theirs too. Due to the very personal nature of the doctor/patient relationship it is impossible for a consultation to develop as it would without a third party there.

What did become obvious to me early on was that my trainer and his patients were on very good terms, more friends than professional and client. The town (t'Brig) was not affluent and some families' circumstances were far less than ideal. Thus, to examine someone's acute abdomen in a cramped, dimly lit room on a bed which sagged badly, surrounded by dogs, children and cigarette smoke, was rather different from bright white sterile hospital examination rooms surrounded by nurses and equipment. I enjoyed getting out and about on house calls from which one could learn a great deal about the physical, psychological and social factors influencing a family. To be out of doors in daylight hours in the working week was wonderful after the claustrophobic hospital environment.

During that year I worked towards my examination to be accepted as a member of the Royal College of General Practitioners. As no doubt with many professional examinations, I found myself drawn into the jargon one used in lectures, tutorials and examinations. 'Perceive learning needs.' 'Explore hopes, fears and expectations.'

To me this was a complicated way of stating the obvious, but I suppose sometimes even the obvious needs to be stated. When helping a family with bereavement, 'Offer sympathy and support.' Examination marks were actually given for writing this. I felt that if one needed to be told to offer sympathy and support after a death, then one shouldn't be in general practice anyway – or, in fact, anything else to do with looking after people. Perhaps, to some, dealing with people does not come naturally.

During this year I also obtained my Diploma of the Royal College of Obstetricians and Gynaecologists. By now I could sign myself Dr Clive Barker MB ChB MRCGP DRCOG. This is not recommended though, as a colleague of mine who also obtained his Diploma in Child Health found when writing to a consultant surgeon, and ending with all 17 letters after his name. The reply came signed with the consultant's name followed by: CLEVER DICK.

We met our peers at what we described as 'playschool' one day a week, which was our general practitioner trainee workshop. Twenty of us would meet to discuss various aspects of general practice. Already there were the embryonic stereotypes of the characters which make up general practitioners, from the earnest bearded 'knit your own yoghurt' type with badly fitting corduroys, elbow pads and sandals, to the clean-cut striped-shirted business types, with more paperwork than medical equipment in their bags.

At that time I carried just about every conceivable drug I could need in my bag. As we had all been worried about the embarrassment of arriving at an emergency only to find the needed drug way out of date, I was already fairly obsessive about checking this would not happen to me. This didn't mean that I wasn't caught out in other ways.

After a little while in practice I was called to see an insulin-dependent diabetic whose blood glucose had gone so low he was having a hypoglycaemic episode where he was semi-conscious, disorientated and involuntarily violent. Luckily, I had my new kit of glucagon – a hormone to rapidly reverse these effects. On snapping open the small box I was pleased to see two small ampoules. I drew up the fluid in one and gave it intramuscularly to my patient. He didn't change. Must need the second vial. I then found out that the first vial contained only the water with which to dilute the second ampoule with which I was left. So now all I had was white powder and no water with which to dilute it. Luckily, I found a good vein through which to inject the alternative treatment, intravenous glucose, to which the patient responded well, as I mumbled some excuse as to why my first treatment hadn't worked.

I got to know the area quite well, in particular the pubs and clubs to which I was frequently called to see someone who had passed out through a variety of medical conditions, as well as a variety of beers and spirits. My training practice also covered the local prison, and on a couple of occasions I had the unenviable task of working out whether an inmate was genuinely ill, or trying to get out.

In fact, deciding whether a patient is mildly, moderately or severely ill, is not as easy as it may initially seem. Some of the most innocuous sounding complaints over the phone can lead one to a desperately ill patient, and conversely some of the most dramatic descriptions of illness can send one dashing to a patient who by the time of arrival looks better than the rushing doctor. Even after a thorough history and examination of the patient, it can sometimes be unclear just how poorly the subject is.

Most GPs find this one of the most taxing areas of the job; deciding when it is appropriate to care for someone at home rather than admit them to hospital can be difficult. The easy thing would be to admit everyone to hospital, but this would not be fair to the patient and their family, or practical for the ambulance service or hospitals. I don't know one general practitioner who has not gone home worrying about a patient they have just seen, and hoping the correct decision has been made.

The most distressing cases in my first year were sudden deaths, particularly one case of 'cot death' or 'sudden infant death syndrome.' I felt totally useless having been called to a babe who was lying lifeless barely an hour after the parents had checked their little one who was breathing normally and sleeping peacefully. I quickly learned that there are sometimes no words or actions that can help, but perhaps at least being there provides a little comfort.

At that time, when on call I had an answerphone for people to leave requests for visits on, and aware that there were some potentially urgent cases, I used to hare around the area as fast as it was safe and practical to do. Finding houses at night can be taxing indeed. I now feel that by law each home should have two-foot high illuminated numbers on the front. Whoever designs the orders of dwellings on new developments should spend a day with a general practitioner or a postman. I quickly learned to take explicit directions, and at night I instructed the caller to turn all the house lights on to give me a chance of actually finding my destination.

One frustrating aspect of on-call work is that when one has actually found the address in question, it can seem to take an inordinately long time for the door to be answered. If within the last hour someone has called for a doctor to visit, I would have thought it was logical for the caller to then anticipate the doctor's arrival. Instead, on a few visits one would imagine that they were expecting an axe murderer to visit, as several chains, bolts and locks need to be undone once the doctor's identity has been established through a conversation that took place from each side of the door. Occasionally people even fall asleep having requested a visit, and I have stood in total darkness and driving rain waiting for the door to be answered. It is then not unusual to walk into a room blue with cigarette-smoke haze, with the TV blaring and various dogs straining to get at this apparent intruder.

On other occasions we can be at fault by arriving at the wrong house. This seems to occur on calls when access is unusually easy. I have at times waited a polite length of time for the door to be answered, and when it has not been, yet it is unlocked, I have walked in only to startle a total stranger who has certainly not called for a doctor.

Another aspect I also began to appreciate gradually at this time was the patient's point of view. It was easy for me to grumble inwardly at inappropriate calls, but I have medical training and most people do not. Reversing a similar situation, at this time I lent my video recorder to my parents, and when I got it back it didn't work. After a brief examination I phoned the engineer who kindly visited. Within seconds he got it working.

'How did you do that?' I enquired.

'I pressed the on/off switch,' he replied, looking like I might look at an unnecessary call. The switch position must have altered in transit and I hadn't figured it out.

Life in my bachelor pad was comfortable enough, but I began to hanker after a little more permanency. I had spent several years moving from one job to another and one place to another. Carole and I were very happy together, and I was not so contented when we were apart, and nor was my stomach. Cooking for one can be a rather sad and lonely experience, and so I attended several postgraduate meetings over that year, with particular interest in the food being served beforehand. One winter evening, I ventured out to a local hotel, more attracted by fulfilling my nutritional rather than my educational needs, and chatted before the meeting to one of the senior local GPs.

I had met one of his partners a few weeks before at a local amateur boxing event. The senior partner in my training practice had been unable to represent Preston as a guest and medical officer at this charity event due to prior commitments, so asked me to go. I duly attended, in requisite dinner jacket, to witness several bouts where enthusiastic youths beat each other up, watched by dozens of mainly drunken guests. Not being a fan of this sport anyway, and the disparity between some of the sparring partners' abilities reminding me of my school sporting days, I vowed never to attend another of these events.

Almost as reluctant to be party to these events, but fortunately more willing to get into the ring to minister to the puny loser splayed out on the mat, Iain was the GP representing Chorley. As we chatted in our ringside seats, hoping not to get blood, sweat or tears in our coffee, I realised we had met before. Iain had been a GP in my home village some years before and, in fact, our first occasion of meeting was over my testicles, which had become swollen due to mumps! Fortunately, neither of us remembered the fact on that evening over dinner, and instead we chatted about life in general practice and in Chorley.

These unplanned meetings with two partners in a local practice were to lead to my arrival in Chorley. At that time I hadn't started in earnest to look for partnerships, and this course of events led me to believe a little more in so-called fate than I had previously done. Some of my at least equally able colleagues had been searching quite frantically for jobs, perhaps because they had more commitments, financially or domestically, yet nothing had arisen. One morning, after surgery in Bamber Bridge, a phone call came through to me from Alex, the senior partner.

'When do you finish?' was his initial brusque question. Taken by surprise I replied, 'About eleven o'clock.'

'No, no, no, when do you finish your trainee year?'

'The end of August.'

'Good,' he said, and then told me he and his partners would like to see me in a few days' time in Chorley.

Before I had the chance to ask anything further, the conversation was over. In fairly relaxed mode I therefore travelled the few miles to their practice, to what I thought was an informal browse around their premises. The secretaries soon made me feel very welcome, and I was then shepherded in to one of the consulting rooms, where I was stunned to see all six partners in the practice were gathered. Rather daunted initially, I was quickly put at my ease while we all chatted about my 'Hopes, fears and expectations', as the Royal College of General Practitioners would put it, of life in general practice.

They seemed an amiable bunch with a sense of humour who obviously had a different approach to seeing prospective partners than some I was hearing about – stories of my contemporaries having to endure interviews where their social graces were more important than their medical ability. At these 'trial by ham salads', a prospective GP's spouse or partner would be invited around for hors d'oeuvres and assessed for their suitability as a member of Rotary or Ladies Circle. I understand these would usually go very badly, with the interviewee walking dog-dirt on to the white shagpile carpet or some similar mishap.

A few days after my visit I was asked back for an interview, so, wearing my rarely worn but rather worn out suit I went again. Within a few minutes I had been offered a place in their partnership, with an initial six months 'mutual assessment' period, and a further two and a half years to full parity. I was very flattered, and as I thought of all the questions we were told to ask of promising practices, most of them had already been answered.

Before I could bring up the sometimes thorny question of practice finances, I was given a complete set of practice accounts to read and to show to my father or other advisers in confidence. In return, they just asked me to let them know when I had decided. Unusually for me, this didn't take very long and, fortunately, in the 10 years since making the decision to accept, I have never regretted it.

As the time to start grew nearer, Alex invited me down again for a chat. He was outwardly rather an intimidating man, who gave me some of the benefit of his 30 years' experience. He told me in serious terms about the commitment and stamina that was needed for a lifetime in general practice. He advised me not to make hasty decisions about house-buying, or to go out and buy a fancy car, as something solid like a Volvo would be a sensible idea in a few months' time. At that point I tried not to peer too obviously out of his blinded window at my shiny new red Ford Escort XR3i purchased within days of being appointed.

He had dedicated himself to general practice, and though outwardly firm and rather autocratic, inwardly he clearly loved his patients and the job. Due to the enormous amount of time he had spent at work, he felt at times that he had missed his children growing up, and told me that I was definitely not to do the same, and that general practice is a way of life but that it is not one's whole life, a fact which I have tried to keep in focus ever since.

In Chorley I would be near to Carole, my parents, and my training practice, as well as the hospitals I had worked in. In fact, I was able to keep my little flat on while we explored the area and looked at places to live. After moving from job to job for the last few years I was pleased to look forward to some stability in my work, and also my finances. I had just about paid off all the money I owed my parents from university days, when I had no money but plenty of time to spend it, but now I had some money but less time. I insisted on repaying their generosity, by giving them an extra one penny more than I had borrowed, so that it could never be said that I had never paid a penny's interest on my loan – not that Mum or Dad would have ever commented. In fact, they lent my brothers and me money even when it took them further into debt. I hope, as I am sure my own children do, that I can be as generous.

CHAPTER SIXTEEN

'I thought I told you to be here at eleven o'clock?' said my senior partner on my first morning, at ten thirty.

I was only trying to be keen, and fortunately our two secretaries took me under their wing and reassured me that this was the norm. The reception staff also seemed friendly, and plied me with a large amount of coffee and encouragement. My huge new shiny leather doctor's bag drew gasps of admiration, as well as the occasional sarcastic comment from one or two of my new partners.

The health centre was crowded with doctors, and I didn't have a surgery of my own at that time. The uninteresting flat-roofed health centre had been built in the early seventies when such places were all the fashion, but due to the already expanding role of the primary health care team, the 16 doctors and their staff were rapidly outgrowing the premises by the time I got there in 1986. A huge impersonal waiting room accommodated all the patients of every practice, all with their coloured numbered plastic cards, which the patients patiently waited with until their number came up. The call system frequently broke down, and the doctors' coloured call lights couldn't be seen to flash when the sun was in a certain direction. Some patients would get even more confused than they already were, and fights would almost break out over whose turn it was to see the doctor!

Our practice operated a personalised list system where patients would be encouraged to see their own doctor wherever possible, and most preferred this for obvious reasons. This led to a little apprehension when people were advised that their own GP was booked up, but that they could see the 'new doctor' if they wished. The new doctor sat there twiddling his thumbs for a large part of the first day or two, and people came in dribs and drabs, some out of curiosity rather than illness. But that was the last time I ever had spare time in all the years since!

I was made most welcome by all the team, and our patients, and many people who consulted in those first few weeks I am still seeing. Perhaps 10 years on I still haven't found what's wrong with them! In fact, I had grandiose ideas that even though some of them had been seeing various different doctors for years, now that I had arrived with a little more time initially to assess their cases, I would surely sort them out. Naive. In later years these same people would move on to subsequent additions to the practice, as I hadn't been able to make the difference to their lives that we had hoped.

Home visits were enjoyable, except when I got lost. The town consists of large numbers of terraced streets, and bungalows or semi-detached houses. A few enormous houses built at the turn of the century bordered the main roads, a legacy of the prosperous mill owners, though many are now rest or nursing homes. Chorley is well served by motorways, and the A6. In fact, it is very easy indeed to leave. Not many folk come to visit, but some call en route elsewhere.

The surrounding villages are attractive little communities, and two or three miles from the centre of the town there are some little hamlets nestling at the foot of the West Pennine Moors. On public holidays I used to zip over the motorway bridges into some beautiful countryside, sparing a glance on the way past to the motorways choked with static traffic on its way to Blackpool or the Lake District.

The town centre has seen better days, though on a Tuesday there is a very busy thriving market. This is fortunate, in that when advertising for new partners we could describe our, 'thriving market town.' Most budding GPs at the time when I applied seemed to want to work in a 'thriving market town.' Perhaps they have read too many books or seen one of the exponentially increasing number of medical dramas on television set in such places. The latter, in fact, usually bear no resemblance to real life in general practice. Our patients seem to get the wrong idea too. According to the portrayals on television we have huge amounts of time to potter around, popping in to see our flock for mainly a friendly chat. If only!

Peak Practice and *Eastenders*, currently popular serials, portray the doctors dropping in for an hour or two at hospitals some miles away, or helping out with the ferreting. I credit my patients with more sense than to think that is an accurate representation, though I wonder sometimes if a few folk think we have time to spare. We do sometimes receive unusual requests for visits, such as one lady recently who had locked herself out of her house and thought we were the most appropriate people to phone, but in the main the requests we receive are reasonable.

My very first evening visit was to see a lady in her seventies whose neighbours thought she was behaving slightly strangely. On arrival I was met by a grey-haired lady who cannot have been much over five-feet tall, who I would probably have taken more kindly to were she not wielding a large carving knife and shouting for me to go away. It transpired this lady had her life savings hidden under her bed, and had become increasingly paranoid about this, to the point of psychosis. After calling the consultant psychiatrist and mental health approved social worker, this lady, who I hoped wasn't too typical of my average patient-to-be, was admitted to hospital.

Fortunately, most of my consultations were somewhat less dramatic. One of the early trials, however, was getting used to certain aspects of the local dialect. Now that I have lived in Lancashire for most of the last 14 years my early BBC accent is broadening. I also now know that 'avin' a road through' means moving one's bowels, and 'kekking over on t'side coaster' means twisting one's ankle on the kerb. Not surprisingly, when first confronted with these phrases I was somewhat puzzled. As ever, folk were gentle with me and patiently explained what the 'eck they were on about! In fact, I can honestly say that I can't imagine a better group of people to work for than Chorley folk. They are honest with me, and I can be honest with them. There is little waffling and skirting around the issues here. Although an alien to Lancashire, at least I was from the North West of England, though I am pretty sure people are made welcome wherever they are from.

When discussing medical practice in Chorley compared to an area which would like to consider itself more affluent, I asked one of my colleagues what they felt the difference was. He replied, 'One of the good things about Chorley is that we are not called to see our partners' private patients in the middle of the night because they happen to be pissed and demand to see a doctor.' In fact, we don't have any private patients, though we do have one or two who like a drink or two.

Ten years on in general practice, I have got to know most of my patients pretty well, and they have got to know me. But in the early years I felt a sense of having to prove myself. While I would never now be complacent,

I do feel comfortable, as most of my patients also seem to be, in the knowledge that I will usually get it right. Back then, I was an unknown quantity both to my patients and to myself. However, I was usually given the benefit of the doubt and only a handful of people would say, 'Well, actually, Doctor X usually gives me this or does that.'

Even if they did give me hints about how they would like to be managed I was only too happy to go along with this usually, as they and their GP had a relationship going back years. Fortunately, my colleagues were and still are of such a calibre that, together in partnership with their patient, they knew what was best.

This was a key issue I discovered in general practice. Whereas in hospital most people in those days expected to be advised or told what was the best course of action, and indeed would sometimes be stunned to be asked what they felt, in general practice courses of management are discussed together before being embarked upon. Older patients did sometimes rather tend to accept without question what 'the doctor' said, though this is not always a wise move. It still surprises me that some of my more senior citizens have large scars in their abdomen where long-retired surgeons have removed various organs or part thereof, and on my enquiring as to what was removed and why, the patient has absolutely no idea. Such trust.

In order to familiarise myself with patients' medical histories, I started summarising their records. Laboriously going through the hospital letters, lab reports, and GP notes, I would piece together the story which made up people's medical lives. At first our notes were not tagged in chronological order, and on seeking out what might be a relevant report, sets of notes would explode all over the desk, a jumble of often unintelligible scrawl.

An interesting feature was that as treatments became more available, the records of consultations would become more lengthy and detailed. As people's expectations increase, and as the threat of complaints and legal action becomes ever more present, GP's notes have got even more comprehensive. Thorough notes, of course, are very important. Practising defensive medicine, where every possible avenue is explored in increasingly detailed, often unpleasant, and sometimes potentially dangerous procedures, to pursue an exceedingly unlikely diagnosis, might not be so good.

After six months in general practice I began to experience a phenomenon I had been warned to watch out for: itchy feet – not, this time, due to rampant athlete's foot. After several years of upping sticks every few months to move on to a new job, sometimes in a new place, it is a strange feeling to think that one might be in the same place for the next 35 years. This can be rather daunting, though on the positive side job security is a huge reassurance. On moaning about the negative aspects of my job, I sometimes need to remind myself that many hundreds of thousands, if not millions, of people in this country alone would be grateful for the job security I have.

My itchy feet soon settled on assessing the other positive aspects of the job at that time. I found that as the months went by, my confidence in the job and myself grew, and this time I wouldn't have to move into a field about which I knew very little. The financial rewards were relatively high in the first few years of general practice. As with most practices at that time, I drew a two-thirds share of income for the first three years, and then a full partnership share, which means I was on my maximum income by the age of 30. My father pointed out that it would be prudent to invest or save some of this for later years, and I am only now realising what sound advice this would have been, had I taken it!

As I began to feel comfortable about my future in general practice, I had the unsettling experience of my first real illness. For a few days at work in the late winter of that first year, I had felt somewhat fluey, taken paracetamol and carried on working. After all, I was a fit, 27-year-old who had never had a day off work. I then started becoming chesty, so I treated myself with a standard antibiotic and kept going. Treating oneself, I found out, is a bad move. Just like treating one's family, it is impossible to be objective, and doctors are known for never taking their own advice anyway.

After a weekend on call I began to feel really ill, and on the Monday morning I started coughing up blood. I sat in surgery feeling worse than my patients until, prompted forcibly by Carole, I decided it was time to seek advice. I was packed off home despite my pleas that I was okay and could carry on. A more potent antibiotic was commenced, and a chest X-ray arranged. I got a slight shock when the radiographers put up the X-ray of a patient with a lung tumour for me to study, but on seeing my colour drain even more, they admitted that was a bad joke, and my X-ray only showed a right middle lobe pneumonia. This was caused by a bug called mycoplasma, confirmed by blood testing. In fact, I even managed to confirm the same way which patient I had caught it from.

I have a collection of cartoons displayed on my surgery wall, which I have collected over the years. One from this episode was a get well card I received. A doctor is sitting about 12 feet from his patient, with an extra long stethoscope, leading from his ears, to her chest. She is sitting up in bed holding the bell end of the stethoscope to her own chest, and he is saying, 'What makes you think it's catching?'

Four weeks later I was fit enough to return to work, with a new insight into what it was like to be ill, and therefore a new sympathy for those patients who also were.

Recuperating from this unpleasant illness made me realise how much I needed Carole, and not just to nurse me. In the spring after my illness, we spent a wonderful two weeks in south-east Spain, doing very little apart from being together. I felt mentally and physically drained and this was an excellent pick-me-up. The summer passed with me feeling closer and closer to the girl I knew I loved. For some reason it took me another few months to propose to her. I imagined that to pluck up courage to do this was a big deal, and that I should deliberate and wrestle with my thoughts about such a major step. In fact, I deliberated so much I wouldn't have been surprised if she had given up on me! It was pretty obvious to everyone else we were set for life.

In the autumn, we spent two weeks in America. The first week was with an old schoolfriend of mine, Andy, who is still working as an accountant in New York where he now has a family. The second week we spent with my brother Alec in Seattle. Alec works for Microsoft, and seemed to be working as many hours as I used to in hospital medicine. I always envied Alec's intelligence, though I would never admit it to him directly, and no doubt his seemingly planet-sized brain helped him tremendously in those relatively early days with that company in the mid 1980s. He had yet to meet his wife-to-be, Terry, and he was obviously lonely. We all felt empty after saying goodbye at the airport after a wonderful week which included activities such as white-water rafting. This was exhilarating indeed, though I wonder if we would be quite so keen now, with dependent children.

Alec and Terry met shortly afterwards, partly through the Microsoft soccer team. They returned to England where they were married, and spent some time in the lovely Derbyshire village of Parwich. They returned to Seattle where Alec works for Microsoft again, and though this spell away from the company means that he is not the millionaire he would have been had he not left, we can see how very much happier, if somewhat more sleep-deprived, he is with Terry and his children Emily and Christopher.

My youngest brother Guy, and his fiancée Anne, also live in Seattle now, having conducted the longest-distance romance I have yet encountered. From what I remember they were briefly training in Nottingham, she in nursing, he in having a good time while pretending to be on an electronic engineering course at university. He was the nearest any of us Barker boys came to the rock star, though still missed by several million light years. I understand the university hall review programmes were distributed to the audience, then rapidly collected up again, as someone realised that his group 'Rectal Discharge' (or 'RD' as he now refers to it) inadvertently appeared on them.

He then travelled south, for a few years in computing, then over to Seattle to work with Alec. Guy now works with Microsoft as an independent contractor, hopefully soon to attain his green card. Anne migrated to New York, same country, different coast, by three thousand miles. Now she is nursing in Seattle so that, at last, after more than 10 years, they are actually in the same city again. Luckily, no 'RD' reunions are planned, because if they were, I would imagine the green card might take a little longer! Seriously, though, I am sure Guy and Anne are both real assets to the communities within which they work.

CHAPTER SEVENTEEN

On returning to England I made up my mind to propose to Carole. The question was *when*. Perhaps in these matters, fate really can play a part because the next week we saw a house that was to become our first home. I had seen it briefly before, but was bleeped for work while halfway through looking around it. I had rather dismissed it, but Carole showed more interest, and her shedding a tear or two looking from the back bedroom over the quiet sheltered garden… I didn't need to ask if this was the one.

That same week Carole left me a note, which I still have, saying, 'Hello dear', but instead of the word 'dear' there was a little drawing of a deer, and several other words were replaced by sweet little drawings. She had gone to work, and as I stood alone in my flat that day I knew absolutely what I wanted to do. I have never been so sure of anything in my life, and that weekend, after all the romantic settings we had seen together, I proposed in my dingy flat by the M61 motorway. It was the easiest thing in the world to do, and thankfully for me Carole said 'Yes'. My only regret is that I hadn't asked sooner.

Seven months later we were married.

We thoroughly enjoyed the lead-up to our wedding. Some people appear to get somewhat harassed about these things but there really is no point in that. Providing the two people who are getting married are right for each other, then surely finishing touches like the weather, the speeches, and how many silly hats are on display, are immaterial.

Carole got an inkling as to how overzealous I am regarding punctuality on our way to our engagement photograph, which was a freebie from the chap we'd booked to photograph our wedding. She was late, or more likely

I was unreasonably early, and we had a minor difference of opinion, which we had not quite resolved by the time we sat looking longingly into each other's eyes in the photographic studio. The photographs came out surprisingly nicely!

As well as organising the wedding, we moved into our new home in the early winter of 1987. Our parents were very tolerant of the fact that we weren't yet actually married, but I don't think the quiet, leafy, 'prime residential area' that we had chosen was used to this state of affairs. I think we set one or two curtains a-fluttering, but in fact everyone was very welcoming, and we were blissfully happy there.

On moving in, the previous occupants had taken the curtains, carpets, light fittings, garden shed, and even one of the toilet seats. The garden was in a beautiful condition, but the decorating left something to be desired, such as the fridge-freezer having been wallpapered around, rather than moved when the room was decorated. Having no enthusiasm or talent for matters DIY, and fortunately having some spare cash at the time, I was happy to employ people to paint, wallpaper, carpet and do all the other tasks that any real man would take on themselves. One of my philosophies in life is to let tradespersons ply their own trades to their best ability, while I do the same in mine, and if necessary work a few extra hours for the on-call service to pay others to do their bit.

I must have still looked fairly young to be lucky enough to own this property, as on one occasion I answered the door to a salesman who asked me if my dad was in! Unfortunately, nobody seems to ask that any more…

By the time our wedding was near, we had a lovely cosy home. We were a long the first of our friends to have a home with a couple of spare bedrooms, so the house was frequently used for weekend get-togethers. What our new neighbours thought about all these young couples coming and going I am not quite sure. We decided not to start trying for a family until a few months after we were married, but some of our friends, worried that they would be subfertile after too many years working and socialising too hard, seemed to have started trying a little early. As it happened some of them weren't as subfertile as they thought, and one or two wedding dates were brought forward over the years, and for all I know some of the resulting offspring could have been conceived in our house. It certainly seems a very fertile home.

We had a full house the weekend of our stag and hen nights. In fact, it appears these days that one evening is not enough, and these celebrations go on at least a weekend. Hence the lads and I went off to play golf very badly, then off to Preston to a few pubs and a pizza restaurant. The first pub we tried to visit had been knocked down, perhaps in anticipation of our arrival, but we had more success elsewhere.

Shortly after arriving at the pizzeria, a policewoman kissogram, organised by Danny, arrived to read out a poem even more full of errors than the first draft of this book, and to the wrong person! Carole and the girls were no doubt having a more civilised time out elsewhere, but we all arranged to meet up in a nightclub frequented by other people such as ourselves who were getting rapidly too old for these nights out. We were dragged up on stage, and when asked if I had anything to say to Carole, I proposed to her again, only to learn later that her ex-boyfriend was also in the nightclub, and I will be eternally grateful to him for not taking exception to this.

Four weeks later (so we could recover from that evening) we all met up again. After a relaxed evening out with Ewan and Karen, Carole and I went our separate ways for the last time, she to her parents' home and I to mine. My best man and I had a couple of nightcaps together and, at a little before midnight, retired. Feeling relaxed and in control I drifted off to sleep, only to be woken a few minutes later by the shrill call of the bedside telephone.

'I bet you're really nervous right now,' or words to that effect, came Brian's voice through my sleepy haze. From that moment I barely slept a wink.

As my wedding day dawned, at around five o'clock in the morning, I stood at the kitchen sink, washing up, thinking of all the friends and family who would be wending their way towards Christ Church in Fulwood for our big day. On that day, Saturday 7 May 1988, the sun never stopped shining. Blossom blew from the trees on what seemed like a light breeze, but which sounds on our wedding video like a Force Eight gale. Hats scattered in all directions and so, in fact, did my nerves, which on arriving at the church were completely forgotten.

What I felt that day truly is indescribable. Nearly all the people we loved and cared about gathered together in that one special place. The next time that might happen could be our funeral, and then there wouldn't be so many, and we wouldn't be there to enjoy it. As Carole walked down the aisle and drew close to me I couldn't help thinking what a sweet nose she has, and how beautiful she looked. Then I couldn't help noticing she was having a supraventricular tachycardia (SVT), as some of her decorative flowers oscillated at about 200 times per minute.

On a few occasions over the previous years she had surprised me by going into this benign but unsettling cardiac arrhythmia. The first time I just thought it was my natural charm that had set her heart a-fluttering, but sadly not.

'She's going to pass out,' I thought. 'Still – no better place than at the altar on our wedding day.' Fortunately, her blood pressure sustained her throughout the ceremony, and to the closing hymn we walked slowly up to the altar. Towards the end of the closing hymn, 'Now Thank We All Our God', I felt a wave of emotion I had never known before. At the risk of sounding embarrassingly sentimental, it is impossible to describe, but I can honestly say that if life's experiences can be measured, then I don't think it would be possible to be more fulfilled and happier than I was at that moment.

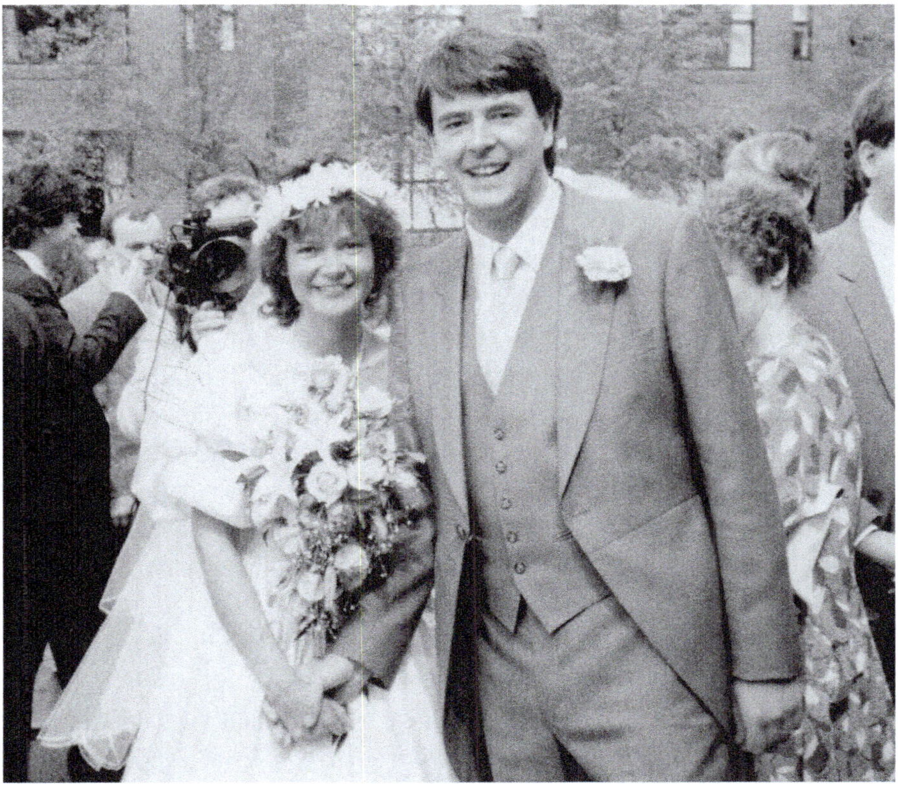

Our wedding day, May 7th 1988

Knowing we wouldn't be having an unplanned reception on the coronary care unit, Carole's SVT having stopped, I relaxed completely for the rest of the day. To be the centre of attention is wonderful, though rather tiring, and it was one of the occasions I felt a little sympathy for some members of the royal family who must spend their whole lives like this.

Towards midnight the guests dispersed, and we retired to our honeymoon suite. Carole looked radiant, and as we lay on our four-poster bed together, all tiredness suddenly forgotten, the phone went. Not my mate again, but my mother-in-law. Before we could explain we could figure out what to do next by ourselves, she told us one of the wedding party had lost her keys, and asked if they were in our room, which had been taken over as a hairdressing salon earlier in the day.

The next morning we were so keen to see everyone we were out first, and had an equally enjoyable and slightly more relaxed day, which ended as we drove home, with a coachload of school kids cheering as we drove down the motorway to our house, with streamers and confetti all over the car.

Three days later we set off for our secret honeymoon destination. Not even Carole knew where we were going. I inadvertently let the cat out of the bag at the airport, though, where we were set to fly to St Lucia in the Caribbean. As it transpired, it was just as well that my new bride did know where we were going, because the novelty of the secret was beginning to wear off as we were delayed several hours at Gatwick Airport. Then we arrived in St Lucia in stifling late evening humidity.

The cramped minibus to the furthest point from the airport on the island, our hotel, induced another SVT as we bumped through all the potholes in the worn road. On arriving at our hotel on this adventure, which had consumed the rest of my savings, we found out our room was as far from reception as it was possible to be and still be in the same resort. Eventually, we made it to our room. I collapsed under the weight of our cases and Carole headed for an essential cooling bath, only to find out there was no cold water.

My everlasting memory of our honeymoon night is of Carole, utterly exhausted, collapsing into one or two inches of hot water in the bath, which I tried to fill with ice cubes from the machine outside our room. I stepped out of our patio window, however, to realise why we hadn't spent two weeks youth-hostelling. After a few yards of soft grass, cool fine sand enveloped my aching feet, and a few yards further on I felt the cool still waters of the Caribbean Sea.

Most other couples were honeymooners, and those who weren't seemed to be celebrating an anniversary. The atmosphere was totally relaxed, and the only anxious people I saw for the whole two weeks were those youngsters who had sneaked out of the UK to secretly get married, without telling any of their families, and after two weeks in paradise were wondering what they were going to tell the folks back home.

By the second day all was well for us, and we had a wonderful two weeks. Only once did I get offered something to expand my mind by one of the locals, but being firmly against any illicit drugs, however 'soft', and having never taken any, I declined. Anyway, I was feeling high on the place, the cocktails and being with Carole, so I didn't need any other help. I hope that those people who welcomed us so warmly to their island would be equally warmly accepted back in England, though I am well aware this isn't always the case. In fact, I did find the colonial attitude of the Caucasian hotel managers towards some of the locals who worked there distinctly unsettling.

All too soon our two weeks were over, and we flew back to the real world. This was to be the last of our long-haul trips for some time. I had given up trying to play the seasoned traveller on a previous occasion where I nonchalantly said to the check-in staff at the airport that if there were seats in first or business class upstairs, then we would be willing to pay a reasonable upgrade fee to be placed there. I had heard that this made journeys on the jumbo jets that I assumed were used for all these routes more palatable. The check-in clerk sneered at me condescendingly and said, 'There is no upstairs on this flight. You would be sitting on the roof.' Since then I have tried to impress Carole many times, and almost always met with abject failure.

CHAPTER EIGHTEEN

Back in the real world I settled again into life in general practice. A working day of eleven or more hours started about seven thirty in the morning with paperwork and then three hours morning surgery during which I would see twenty to twenty-five patients. The time for each consultation used to be five to seven minutes for most GPs, but this has increased to nearer eight or ten minutes for most of us, as it is difficult to address someone's problems properly in less than this. In fact, most doctors and patients would rightly argue that ten minutes is too little, but with an ever-increasing demand it would be impossible to see everyone who felt they needed to consult in a day, if one took longer.

In the late morning I would set off for my house calls and it was not unusual to make eight or ten visits, though this number has decreased for most GPs in recent years. I used to enjoy this traditional part of practice life, when one could glean information about a patient's social and family circumstances, and seem more a part of a community myself. People seemed to appreciate house calls, and I am well aware that they are missed by our patients. However, as two or three people can be seen at surgery in the time it takes to make one house call, the latter is not an efficient use of doctors' time. This may sound harsh as it can be an inconvenience for many patients, and sometimes practically not easy, but unless visits are restricted to those people for whom it is genuinely difficult to go out, we wouldn't complete our day's work until midnight.

In years gone by I would be asked to see patients at home, at a specific time, as they were going out later to the hairdressers or the shops! My predecessor used to visit a huge number of chronically ill or disabled people at home and write their prescriptions. Some of these people would then go out themselves to have them dispensed. His day was so full he would start even earlier than I, often finishing later.

One visit I made shortly after he retired, to a rather grumpy elderly lady some miles from our practice, made me vow not to encourage a doctor-dependent population. On arriving at her house, I politely enquired how I could help her, and after mumbling her dissatisfaction that I was not her usual doctor, she told me she needed her prescription. I obliged, and explained that due to my increasing workload, while I would be happy to visit if she needed me for a medical reason, if she only needed her prescription then she could post her card or ask someone to drop it in at the surgery. She was most unimpressed by this and then asked, ‘Does that mean Doctor ... Doctor ... oh, what’s his name, will not be visiting any more?’ After calling every month for over 10 years she couldn’t even remember his name.

A second lesson I learned from such experiences was that though we flatter ourselves to think we are indispensable, doctors are not. Most people might be concerned for our welfare, but they are more concerned, rightly so, for their own, and someone else can pick up where we left off.

Nowadays, I perform between two and five visits per day on average, and even this is more than many GPs. On returning from visits, hopefully grabbing a few minutes for lunch along the way, I start more paperwork, including medical reports, letters (reading, dictating and signing), and updating computer information. Our computer arrived at the end of the 1980s, and though it seemed an intrusion initially, it is now indispensable.

The evening surgery hasn’t changed much in recent years, starting a little after three and going on till six thirty, followed if needed by any late requests for visits. During the afternoon, therefore, another 20 to 25 patients will be seen, meaning that by home time I have attempted to solve 50 or more people’s problems, medical and otherwise. In addition there are numerous phone calls for advice and information. The number of patients seen hasn’t changed much, though there is a huge amount more paperwork, which is almost as boring to write about as it is to do, so I will refrain.

Prior to my years in general practice, my predecessors would often work later into the evening, and perform even more house calls, as transport for patients was not as widely available. There were, however, fewer treatments to contend with, and expectations weren’t quite as high. There was also much less bureaucracy.

It wasn't too many years prior to my arrival that the partners were on call every night for their own patients, meaning that their sleep would be disturbed regularly, though night visits were less frequently requested at that time. Most GPs then organised rotas within their own practice such that they were only on call one or two nights a week and, around the time I arrived, our practice was involved in setting up a medical co-operative. This is an organisation run and staffed by local GPs, as well as telephonists and navigators, which works with basically a large rota, where one works for a defined shift for a few hours, covering a large number of patients.

This means that when one is on call for the co-operative, it is busy, but that one doesn't have to be on call that often. This is preferable to doing only two or three calls from home in an eight- or twelve-hour period. Just like in hospital days it always seemed that the requests for consultations come in at the most inconvenient times, including when just about to eat, go to the toilet or go to bed.

After too many years, the Government is at last realising how deep-seated the feeling is among general practitioners that a 24-hour commitment for every GP is just not possible. At last some funding has been found to help co-operatives similar to ours set up.

Again, after much constructive criticism from us, some aspects of the general medical practitioners' contracts which were imposed in 1990 are being reworked. At last a 'patients not paper' campaign has started, in order to hopefully reverse the trend where GPs and their hardworking staff were spending increasing amounts of their time filling in pointless pieces of paper, instead of helping patients.

In the last few years, other tasks have been forced on us, such as the collection of huge amounts of meaningless data about people's health habits. Many people have no doubt been surprised when they have walked into their doctor's surgery, to find that instead of the problem with which they had intended to consult being addressed, they have been asked how much exercise they take, and whether any close relatives have ever had a stroke. Relevant with certain people though this may be, it rather detracts from the point with most people. This data was needed for a badly thought-out health promotion scheme, which was not effectively evaluated before being introduced throughout all practices.

I put forward our health promotion package as enthusiastically as I could, trying to enter into the spirit of the task, and was awarded a little gold star stuck on my project, as I would have done had I still been in junior school, by an ex-nurse who had become an administrator for the Family Health Services Authority. The first scheme nationally ran for three years, then this was scrapped and another equally silly one ran for another three years, and at last this has been dramatically modified.

It will no doubt become apparent that I have become somewhat disillusioned with certain aspects of general practice. I dearly love the job and my patients, but the way it is being organised by politicians, through administrators, makes me seethe at times.

Two years ago, Carole and I wrote to the prime minister about some of these points, including the exponentially increasing amount of NHS money that was being spent on administrators and managers, while in some areas the amount being spent directly on patients was being cut. We also expressed our unhappiness about some consequences of the charters being introduced. At times these unrealistically and unfairly raise people's expectations of what a hospital or practice could offer, when there was neither the time nor money to back the promises made in practice. We brought up many other points too laborious to go into here, but, to be fair, we received a lengthy and detailed reply addressing each of our concerns.

Ironically, the reply came from someone in an office miles away from the practicalities of everyday medicine and nursing, from the brand spanking new £55 million pound NHS Management Executive building in Leeds. This building was exactly the kind of place we were complaining about, having recently been cited as wasting large amounts of taxpayers' money on expensive carpeting and furnishings.

However, I digress, and must apologise for rambling, but the National Health Service is something I feel deeply about, and something I feel strongly that we must support.

CHAPTER NINETEEN

Family planning is a large and important part of general medical practice, yet most doctors I know are lackadaisical in the organisation of their own families. As with many areas of our work, we tend to concur that, 'A signpost merely points the way, it doesn't actually go down the path.' However, I am sure the members of the medical profession are not alone in being poor takers of their own advice. In fact, when I was spotted at the local garage buying an egg mayonnaise sandwich and pint of banana milk for lunch by a patient of mine who was a local vicar, he opined that this was not a very good advertisement for health. I agreed, but joked that my motto was, 'Do as I say, not do as I do.' He replied, 'What a coincidence, that's my motto too.'

In medicine and nursing we deal with subfertility and infertility a great deal, which can be very rewarding. In fact, in a career where the joyous events are outnumbered by the upsetting, it is a delightful moment when a couple who have had difficulties conceiving attend surgery with a positive pregnancy test, or their first baby. Considering we often have little to do with events, gratitude is sometimes heaped on us to the extent that we feel we have actually been part of a conception.

Most of us end up fairly neurotic that we won't be able to have children. Not Carole and I, however. We were totally cool. We decided to try for a family after a few months of marriage and see what happened, knowing that conception usually takes a few months to occur in one's late twenties or early thirties.

After one unsuccessful month I forgot this, and was convinced we could never have kids. I felt rather pathetic the following month having my early morning bath (without which I can't wake up) and holding my scrotum out of the water to keep the temperature of my gonads down, to aid fertility. Still, it worked, as early one winter morning in 1988 the little indicator on our pregnancy test turned pink and, sure enough, within weeks, Carole was throwing up regularly and looking slightly less radiant than the girl I married only months before.

My general rule is that the more couples have to do with medicine and midwifery, the more complicated are their obstetrics and gynaecological problems. On using the term 'couple' I realise this is a pathetic attempt to indicate I tried to share some of Carole's experiences. I certainly did not share the same appetite. Although I can eat most things, including live fish, Carole's diet of cockles or raw tripe, followed by Mars bars, was more than even I could watch.

In late spring we had a holiday and went to Jersey when Carole was 32 weeks pregnant. Once I knew where the hospital was I was happy and could relax. For the last time we stayed in a hotel where children weren't catered for, and we hired a convertible Ford Escort XR3. We drove to small secluded beaches where we looked forward to the future with hope, excitement and a little anxiety. As we sat on a dry rock miles from anywhere, the only people on the beach, I told Carole how wonderful it was to be alone together for a while. At that exact moment a large prod was felt from Carole's bump, and we knew already that we were not alone.

As it happened we need not have worried about the baby arriving early, as Carole was induced several days overdue as her weight was falling. In the seven years since then, we have stopped weighing ladies in pregnancy in most cases, as it is a poor indicator of foetal and maternal well-being. Perhaps she was induced as people start to get rather jittery a few days after the due date, particularly if the parents are doctors and midwives.

I left Carole at the maternity unit on the evening of 5 July 1989 and sat at home, praying that she and our baby would be okay, and that I would not embarrass myself by trying to interfere or by passing out. A beer and a whisky (which I don't usually drink) later, I lay in bed and dozed off for 10 minutes, after which I was awoken by the telephone. Carole had started in labour, could I come? On arrival she looked slightly less composed than I had last seen her, hyperventilating into an Entonox mask and groaning intermittently.

Sometime before Carole was due, we had asked a midwife who was special to us, having both worked with her and got to know her, if she would

CHAPTER NINETEEN

Family planning is a large and important part of general medical practice, yet most doctors I know are lackadaisical in the organisation of their own families. As with many areas of our work, we tend to concur that, 'A sign-post merely points the way, it doesn't actually go down the path.' However, I am sure the members of the medical profession are not alone in being poor takers of their own advice. In fact, when I was spotted at the local garage buying an egg mayonnaise sandwich and pint of banana milk for lunch by a patient of mine who was a local vicar, he opined that this was not a very good advertisement for health. I agreed, but joked that my motto was, 'Do as I say, not do as I do.' He replied, 'What a coincidence, that's my motto too.'

In medicine and nursing we deal with subfertility and infertility a great deal, which can be very rewarding. In fact, in a career where the joyous events are outnumbered by the upsetting, it is a delightful moment when a couple who have had difficulties conceiving attend surgery with a positive pregnancy test, or their first baby. Considering we often have little to do with events, gratitude is sometimes heaped on us to the extent that we feel we have actually been part of a conception.

Most of us end up fairly neurotic that we won't be able to have children. Not Carole and I, however. We were totally cool. We decided to try for a family after a few months of marriage and see what happened, knowing that conception usually takes a few months to occur in one's late twenties or early thirties.

After one unsuccessful month I forgot this, and was convinced we could never have kids. I felt rather pathetic the following month having my early morning bath (without which I can't wake up) and holding my scrotum out of the water to keep the temperature of my gonads down, to aid fertility.

Still, it worked, as early one winter morning in 1988 the little indicator on our pregnancy test turned pink and, sure enough, within weeks, Carole was throwing up regularly and looking slightly less radiant than the girl I married only months before.

My general rule is that the more couples have to do with medicine and midwifery, the more complicated are their obstetrics and gynaecological problems. On using the term 'couple' I realise this is a pathetic attempt to indicate I tried to share some of Carole's experiences. I certainly did not share the same appetite. Although I can eat most things, including live fish, Carole's diet of cockles or raw tripe, followed by Mars bars, was more than even I could watch.

In late spring we had a holiday and went to Jersey when Carole was 32 weeks pregnant. Once I knew where the hospital was I was happy and could relax. For the last time we stayed in a hotel where children weren't catered for, and we hired a convertible Ford Escort XR3. We drove to small secluded beaches where we looked forward to the future with hope, excitement and a little anxiety. As we sat on a dry rock miles from anywhere, the only people on the beach, I told Carole how wonderful it was to be alone together for a while. At that exact moment a large prod was felt from Carole's bump, and we knew already that we were not alone.

As it happened we need not have worried about the baby arriving early, as Carole was induced several days overdue as her weight was falling. In the seven years since then, we have stopped weighing ladies in pregnancy in most cases, as it is a poor indicator of foetal and maternal well-being. Perhaps she was induced as people start to get rather jittery a few days after the due date, particularly if the parents are doctors and midwives.

I left Carole at the maternity unit on the evening of 5 July 1989 and sat at home, praying that she and our baby would be okay, and that I would not embarrass myself by trying to interfere or by passing out. A beer and a whisky (which I don't usually drink) later, I lay in bed and dozed off for 10 minutes, after which I was awoken by the telephone. Carole had started in labour, could I come? On arrival she looked slightly less composed than I had last seen her, hyperventilating into an Entonox mask and groaning intermittently.

Sometime before Carole was due, we had asked a midwife who was special to us, having both worked with her and got to know her, if she would be willing to deliver Carole.

Without wishing to sound too trendy, since having a baby is such an immensely personal event, we wanted Anne to be involved if at all possible, though of course we were lucky to be helped by many of her very able colleagues too. Thus after working the day already, she arrived in the middle of the night, and Carole still says that as soon as her cold hands touched Carole's warm ones, she knew everything would be all right – and it was. The anaesthetist, of course, couldn't site the epidural first time as, again, is the case when your patient is a midwife, and her anxious GP husband is looking on.

All through the night Carole laboured, the dawn arriving with a large red sun at four in the morning. I remember looking out of the window on the third floor of the maternity block, wondering how we would feel when that sun later set on this day which would change my life more than any other day.

Another six hours later and Carole felt she would never see any other day, as Baby was not for being pushed out. The foetal heart rate began to drop, forceps were being mentioned, but spurred on more than anything by the thought of a bacon butty before the canteen shut at ten thirty in the morning, Carole kept at it. At ten thirty-five, which meant I had to eat the bacon butty, Tom made his appearance into the world. Facing the wrong way around, which explained why progress had been at times agonisingly slow, with a wet blue head and enormous lips, he burst into the world with a croaky cry at 8lb 10oz. So much for the poor weight gain.

I nearly received the injection Carole was supposed to have to prevent haemorrhage as, overcome with emotion, I leaned forward to embrace her. She had told me earlier I was to stay at her head end during the delivery, but I had migrated down to see what was going on, and eventually was a body to push on. After a few minutes with Carole, Tom was laid in his cot, watched over by me in amazement, but also to check he was still breathing, perhaps scarcely able to believe our good fortune in having a chunky, healthy baby.

Carole was not quite so fortunate, having a postpartum haemorrhage there and then, requiring a blood transfusion later on, as her colour was difficult to distinguish from the off-white walls around her. Subsequently, she had two further postpartum haemorrhages requiring re-admission to hospital. Tom also was re-admitted with her, as there was no way she would be separated from him, which would have been practically difficult anyway as she was breastfeeding. He, however, was hale and hearty and has never looked back.

I knew being a dad would change me, both at and away from work, but I couldn't have known how much. The last patient I saw prior to becoming a father was a little boy who, from the description I received over the telephone, might have had meningitis. On arriving at the house it was difficult to examine him to assess this, as he kept hysterically running into the garden. I felt quite sure he did not have meningitis, but I can now better understand the worry parents have about their children. The day after Tom was born I called to see one of my chaps who had just retired, only to have inoperable liver cancer diagnosed. He and his wife unselfishly wished me well with our new arrival as, yet again, I was reminded of our mortality – as one arrives into the world another leaves.

On a happier note, we were inundated with well-wishers. Although not usually a counter of cards, I just had to tot up our new arrival cards. One hundred and fifty, which proves that many other people thought we couldn't manage it either. I even had a caller at our house at eleven o'clock the night Tom was born, who on wishing us well also enquired if he could have something for his wife's piles. I felt the timing of this a little unfair, but gave him some tablets anyway.

CHAPTER TWENTY

After a very special couple of weeks' holiday it was back to work again, to a particularly busy period. Not good timing. My senior partner was retiring after over 30 years in practice. By this time I had acquired several hundred patients on my own list, and many more who had adopted me. Alex seemed to have told most of his 2500 patients that I was taking over from him whereas, in fact, only about half that number were officially transferred to my list. That didn't put them off though, so I was swamped with about 4000 patients all of whom considered me as their doctor.

While initially flattering, I soon realised I just couldn't cope, booked up way in advance and not able to give a good service. Fortunately, I was able to explain to many that they should see my equally, if not more, able and dedicated partners. Thus the workload settled to my current list of about 2400 official patients, the national average being a little under 2000 per doctor.

Since then, I have regularly seen over 200 patients in a week, and up to 70 in a day. We did take on another partner, shortly followed by an eighth, though by mutual agreement initially she worked a two-thirds duty.

I likened my care of patients at that time to keeping plates spinning, as I ran around from one to another trying to keep everyone going. I found myself chasing up people who couldn't be bothered to attend surgery, and following up others on review visits and appointments more frequently than necessary. I began to worry more than I had previously, and it took longer for me to wind down. If not working at a weekend, it would get towards the middle of Saturday before I would relax. I seem to have a need to get on well with people, and at that time I would dwell on consultations which hadn't gone well. Considering I perform many thousands of face-to-face consultations each year, I now accept that a few might not go as well as I would like, or might be difficult.

I recall seeing a lady who was one of my partners' patients, but who chose to see me, possibly as I was weaker, and would accede to her increasingly unreasonable demands to be seen when she wanted for however long she deemed necessary. In the end I was requesting chaperones during the consultation in case of arguments, and as this was clearly an unsatisfactory arrangement we requested she register elsewhere. I deeply dislike removing patients from our list, and must have done so on a total of only 10 occasions or so in 10 years, but at times the doctor/patient relationship irreversibly breaks down.

This, in fact, caused me so much worry that on New Year's Eve at the turn of the decade I thought I had better let matters bother me less, otherwise I would still be worrying about the same cases at the turn of the next decade. Warning bells should have started ringing then, perhaps. I made increasingly copious notes in patients' records, and in my work diary recorded all sorts of work-related matters, just to be on the safe side, to check I had covered everything. I would check and double-check reports just to confirm I hadn't missed anything. Being thorough is a good thing, but being obsessional is not.

I did, however, thoroughly enjoy my work, and found it immensely satisfying, the good spells outnumbering the bad. Many people put up with great physical and mental hardship with stoicism which has to be admired. Many tolerate conditions perhaps not life-threatening, but which significantly impair their quality of life, and complain very little. When I moan inwardly at some of the inappropriate consultations or out of hours visits, I remind myself that there are thousands of others coping with their illnesses alone at home. Sometimes what we provide in the Primary Health Care Team is woefully inadequate, yet those with most to complain about seldom do. Conversely, some of those with the least to trouble them, and for whom we bend over backwards, are only grudgingly, or not at all, appreciative.

When listening to those less satisfied, I try to remember the majority who kindly appreciate what we do. I don't make a habit of keeping letters, but I used to keep a handful to cheer me up at low moments.

'Words seem inadequate, but I know that you certainly saved my life and for that I am and will be eternally grateful to you.' An exact quote from a man in his forties, with a young family, who had a heart attack. Self-congratulatory to keep it I suppose, but we all need that sometimes. Without wishing to appear full of self-importance, there can't be many walks of life where one receives such accolades, and I have treasured selfishly such moments.

At times we do make a difference, when a correct diagnosis or compliment can make one punch the air and quietly say, 'Yes.' Perhaps accountancy or banking can do the same for people, I just don't know.

CHAPTER TWENTY-ONE

So happy were we with Tom, that when he was a year old we thought we would have another go, and bingo, Carole was pregnant again. This time all went well until New Year's Eve 1990, when Carole went to work and ended up as a patient with pain and bleeding.

A scan showed that at twenty-four weeks of pregnancy, the placenta was low-lying. In a grading of seriousness from at best one, to at worst four, this was placenta praevia grade three to four. If it were not for ultrasound scans and caesarean sections, she and the babe would have bled to death in labour. An elective caesarean section was planned for 37 to 38 weeks of pregnancy. Perhaps some obstetricians would have insisted Carole stayed in hospital but, fortunately for us, Mr Wright allowed Carole home, to return immediately should any signs of labour or bleeding ensue. To stay in bed in hospital for over ten weeks, missing her one-year-old son and hopefully me, would have been dreadful, though admittedly a torrential haemorrhage would have been worse.

I tried to remind Carole of this fact when, two days before her planned admission, she started with pains. She lay in a bath at home saying that they would pass. They did, in fact, but if I die prematurely then the damage that day did to my health is surely to blame.

On 2 April 1991 Adam was born. To know that a little after nine in the morning that day our baby was to be born took a lot of the stress out of the event for me. It is not without considerably increased risk to mum, however, but there was absolutely no choice in this case, and as Mr Wright lifted Adam over the green surgical sheet to wave at us, my heart leapt again.

Not to be outdone regarding complications, the day after he and Carole were discharged home, she suffered an SVT which wouldn't stop. Our neighbour came to help out, not for the first time, while Carole and I were whisked off to hospital in an ambulance. This had happened once during the time Adam was expected, and Carole ended up on coronary care, where she was given a low calorie diet and where everyone focussed on her heart, and totally forgot the developing baby.

As patients in neighbouring beds had X-rays and other investigations not wholly conducive to the good health of a pregnant lady, Carole reminded them of her situation. This demonstrates how hospitals can focus on one organ or system rather than the whole patient or, in this case, patients.

Consequently, this second time, Carole was absolutely adamant she would not be admitted to hospital, and even to get her in the ambulance I had to promise I wouldn't let that happen. In hospital she required intravenous administration of a powerful drug with potentially dangerous side effects to stop her cardiac arrhythmia. The medical SHO quite reasonably advised admission for observation overnight. He had coped admirably after what he must have thought was a bad joke: the admission of a senior special care baby unit sister seven days postnatally with an SVT, accompanied by her GP husband.

At Carole's refusal to stay in, however, he turned to me with a sickly pleading smile as if to ask me to sort the situation out. I mumbled to Carole that perhaps it would, after all, be a good idea to stay in. She gave me a look that I still remember and said, 'You've let me down.'

I felt about a foot small, but my concern was for her and that overrode any guilt I felt about breaking a promise.

As it transpired, she was admitted to a ward full of chronic bronchitics, where the dangers to her and Adam were far greater than any from her condition or its treatment, so all agreed she should be discharged. Hence she left hospital vowing never to return, our family seemingly complete to us at that time.

We must have known that it wasn't, as neither of us felt we should go ahead and arrange for anything permanent to be done to us. Adam developed into a beautiful blond blue-eyed boy who was a little rascal from his early months. Yes, it is genetically possible to have a child with such features when both parents have brown eyes and dark hair. We were truly lucky to have two adorable children, jobs we both enjoyed which allowed us to live comfortable lives, and each other, our families and friends to spend time with.

We saw and still see my housemates from university days. Those friendships were made to last. Perhaps we were more similar than we realised. We all became general practitioners, married midwives, and had kids. One of my other friends even suggested we changed cars in unison too.

Our parents have always been of immense help in times when a couple of pairs of extra hands were needed, and Carole's younger sister Joanne has been invaluable, providing emotional and practical support. Pretentious though it sounds, we also have a part-time nanny, Jane, who is another member of our family, totally reliable and dependable, and who allows us to live the full and fulfilled life we do.

I can only guess how younger couples or single parents cope with the demands of work and young children. Admittedly, our vocations can be testing, but we do have support when needed, most of all from each other. When I have had a bad or busy day, I can wind down with Carole, who understands the special demands of such vocations, and hopefully I understand hers when she needs me. Although doctors and nurses are a cliché, it isn't just chance that such people find themselves partners for life.

CHAPTER TWENTY-TWO

One cold wet afternoon my bleep called me to see a man who had felt unwell at work, so had come home. After visiting him, and taking his medical history and examining him, I was confident that he had a viral infection and advised accordingly. To check all was well, I arranged to telephone that evening. An hour later, however, I was called back to see him as he had collapsed. On my arrival he was dead. His wife and the ambulance crew had tried to revive him, in vain, and by the time I arrived he was clearly beyond help.

With a sickening feeling running through me I wondered how on earth this could have happened. The coroner's officer was informed and after some time at the house I then had to go back to surgery and see about 25 people while still in a daze. I did the best I could, and then went back to the house to see how his wife and children were, and then it hit me even more. These kids now had no dad. They looked up at me and I had no answers. I checked them out and checked with the local hospital that there was no obscure condition affecting people in this area, and said I would come back the next day. His wife and family were understanding, knowing that occasionally these events are totally unpredictable in spite of thorough medical assessment.

My partners and I tried to be as supportive to his family as possible and, working together, everyone seemed to get through, apart, of course, from the poor man whose kids knew he had gone to Jesus.

It sounds selfish to describe how I felt, but I thought I was okay, until some months later I began to dwell on how I was able to spend happy times with my family, but he couldn't with his. They would miss him, and perhaps if I had acted differently he could be with them. Admittedly, I would have had to be able to predict the future which, of course, none of us could do, but I still felt guilty. By the next Christmas I was going over and over events again and again. I started writing my thoughts down. I had never been so wrong with a diagnosis before, and I had to justify to myself why I hadn't got it right that time.

Another fact which hadn't helped was that the notes I made on attending him initially got rained on when leaving the house, so I made an exact copy, keeping the original as well, but then wondered if anyone might think I was trying to cover something up. I went to church for comfort, and in the sermon heard the tale where Cain kills Abel, and further bizarre thoughts followed. If I was a decent doctor I would have saved him. I started feeling I was a murderer for not doing.

Writing this now, I realise how disturbed my thought processes were, but obsessional thoughts are very powerful indeed. I spent more and more time ruminating, such that a year after the event I could think literally of nothing else. I then worried in case I accidentally wrote some of these strange thoughts down when supposedly concentrating on something else. I was spiralling down into a situation I could not get out of. In my work diary I was writing to such lengths that one of my colleagues since described it as, '*War and Peace*.'

My own GP and other partners were a great support, but by that time I was in tears at the end of surgeries. I felt I wasn't worthy to treat anyone. I couldn't eat, and lost one and a half stones. I couldn't sleep and started taking sleeping tablets. Panic attacks followed for which I took beta blockers. Then early morning wakening, a cardinal sign of the secondary depression that had set in, where I would suddenly wake, in tears, heart thumping, covered in sweat.

The thoughts wouldn't go away. Every waking minute of every day. The only time I got relief was when the metallic taste of the sleeping tablets would herald a few peaceful hours' sleep. Carole was incredibly patient as I went over and over my worries again and again. I felt my brain was just grinding to a halt, and that I had to stop soon, as I wasn't doing my patients or my colleagues justice. I couldn't ever see myself feeling different or see a way out.

I then saw a consultant psychiatrist who, at very short notice, spent as long as it took for me to tell my sorry tale. It was he who first diagnosed that I had an obsessional condition which had become so bad I had become clinically depressed. He started me on an anti-depressant which, for the first few days, made me feel jaded, dry-mouthed and dizzy. This was particularly embarrassing on trying to fit a coil on a lady, after which I stood up and promptly passed out. I spilt another patient's urine sample all over me because I was trembling so much. Shortly after that I ground to a halt.

Work was impossible. Treatment takes a while to have an effect, and this plus the initial side effects made me stop. At this point I didn't even want to be left on my own. Carole couldn't go shopping or to work without me feeling panicky. Such was the previously confident man whose patients came to him to sort out their problems.

Four weeks passed, during which all sorts of rumours abounded, such as my heart attack, divorce, and others. In fact, I sat at home desperately trying not to think about what had gone before. Sometimes, however, trying *not* to think something means one thinks it all the more! I couldn't even change Adam's nappy at one time without feeling a total lack of self-worth.

As time went by, every now and then a little glimmer of light at the end of the tunnel would appear. I managed to read a short column in a newspaper without obsessional thoughts creeping in. I spent a while gardening, and I began to sleep better. Slowly, my appetite came back and, even more slowly, my confidence crept back. I restarted work, gradually at first, and after seven to eight weeks was back almost to full strength. This was only possible with continuing support from Carole and our families, my friends and colleagues, and the outstanding psychiatric help I received.

I learned a massive amount from this experience. We are not all perfect. We can't get it right all the time. I had tried to be watertight in everything I did, but we can only do our best. I still feel deep sorrow for a good man who is no longer with us, but I don't think any other doctor would have done anything differently.

In our training, we were not taught how to deal with being wrong, or to admit defeat, to be fallible. Doctors have committed suicide worrying about their failures. Though I never got desperate enough to consider this, partly as I thought at the time I was too much of a wimp even to do that, I do remember leafing through my work insurance policies thinking I would never work again. Depression is awful. The stigma of mental illness should not exist. It is as real and at least as bad as physical illness.

Having gone through this I am stronger than I ever would have been. I had a slight relapse some time later, after stopping my treatment too abruptly, coupled with possible overwork trying to re-prove myself, and worry over a partnership split, but since then all I want to do is repay some of the care and knowledge that I have gained in recent years.

CHAPTER TWENTY-THREE

The expanding role of the primary health care team in the early nineties meant that we were outgrowing the increasingly cramped health centre from which we and several other doctors and their staff worked. In order to gain more autonomy over the control of our premises, and to improve our working environment and our patients' facilities, my partners had been looking for alternative accommodation even before I arrived.

The old Chorley library, built at the turn of the century, had been empty for six years when it was advertised for sale. It occupied quite a large site in the middle of Chorley. We had a good look around, to see wet and dry rot, rising and falling damp, and lots of broken glass. An impressive building in its day, and part of Chorley's history, it was unrenovatable. With the help of an architect skilled in these matters, we designed a new purpose-built surgery for our partnership and submitted it for planning approval to the council. We deliberated for hours over how much to bid for the site and, after putting in an offer, worked out to the penny, we were awarded the sale.

We were very pleased with ourselves, until we found out that we had been the only bidders! The old library was taken apart, with some regrets from us and other locals, and the site cleared. Over the following months we saw our new working home take shape, representing many hours planning and several hundred thousand pounds of investment.

Unfortunately, during this time, the two partners who had joined after me, decided to leave. This was not due to the building, but due to a difference of opinions as to the way the partnership worked. In any general medical practice, as with many such groups, the most important factor deciding how the practice runs is whether the partners can communicate and compromise. Due to a number of factors, this did not happen, and they left. Unfortunately, some of us who remained were naive enough to think that partnership separations could be dealt with amicably, and in overzealous efforts to be fair to all parties, the main partnership was left understaffed, and financially disadvantaged. However, due to the fact that we had hard-working and self-sacrificing staff remaining, and because we were lucky to have an excellent doctor to replace those who left, the practice is now stronger than ever.

The partners appreciate that quality of working life is at least as important as financial reward. As for the two who left, their partnership split again within months. I am fiercely loyal to my partners, our staff, and our patients, who together make a damn good team in 'Library House Surgery'.

After two years nurturing our new home, we opened to ... total chaos! The waiting room was too small. Monday morning: seven doctors and two nurses all in surgery at the same time, running late due to technical teething problems. One of my first patients told me, 'I don't know who designed this bloody place but they need to see a doctor.' Resisting the urge to blow a fuse, I explained that we were getting organised and, sure enough, within a week or two we did. We made sure we ran better to time, and staggered various surgeries slightly, as well as enlarging the waiting room by replacing the children's play area with seats, as all the toys disappeared in the first week anyway!

The official opening was by the granddaughter of the original benefactor of the library. It was only right to invite those managers from the Family Health Services Authority who helped us both organisationally and financially in the setting up of the new premises to our opening bash. However, while I was trying to make polite conversation to an FHSA manager, he rather stunned me by saying, 'Well, we could swap platitudes all day. If it doesn't work you could always turn it into a restaurant.'

Fortunately, it is working well.

I don't think we were flavour of the month with the powers that be, as we did not go 'fundholding'. While in favour of more control of our destiny, we have tried to influence purchasing of health care by commissioning groups, rather than fundholding our own single practice budget. None of us want to sacrifice time with patients, to organise lots of small short-term contracts with lots of different providers, seemingly involving disproportionate amounts of time and money in administration. I realise that some would call this naive, and it has been said that one GP with a cheque book is worth 10 in commissioning groups.

Settled in our new building we have built on our stability. Child health surveillance is something I have an interest in, even though I usually have a splitting headache by the end of a two-hour baby clinic, during which I am often urinated and vomited upon – by the children, that is. Diabetic clinics, antenatal clinics, well-woman clinics, hormone replacement therapy clinics, minor operations, as well as dieticians, psychologists, health visitors and district nurses make it a bustling place. I did consider applying to become a trainer in general practice, but at present I just do not have the time necessary.

We also have a large extension to Chorley and South Ribble District Hospital, to which several new consultants have been appointed and, to my horror, some of them are younger than I am. However, this makes me feel less intimidated by my hospital colleagues than I used to, and I look forward to building closer relations.

The mid 1990s are a very exciting time in general practice. The idea of a primary-care led NHS is maturing into a reality. More important is co-operation between the various facets making up the NHS. Perhaps the most important teamwork is between patients and health care staff, each realising the other's capabilities and expectations. To some extent, 'charters' have helped explain what is reasonable to expect in various areas. Unfortunately, they have also sometimes set unrealistic goals, and encouraged a mentality that someone has to be to blame when something goes wrong. This seems to be nurtured by some members of the legal profession, who are now encouraging people to sue their carers when matters do not go well. Of course, it is important to have recourse to complaint, explanation, and compensation, when one is concerned that more could have been done for a patient.

Perhaps the new general-practice based complaints procedure will be better for all concerned, encouraging practice-based informal conciliation where possible. This new system was recently introduced after a review, prompted by the stress recognised to be occurring to all concerned, and in particular by the suicide of one young GP father of four worried about a long protracted complaints procedure.

I do realise that I am viewing these matters from my experience as a medical practitioner, and that, as in every walk of life, there are practitioners not giving the service those who rely on them deserve, and all efforts should be made to rectify that. While trying not to be biased in my discussions in this work, I am merely describing matters how I see them, and I realise others may hold differing views.

CHAPTER TWENTY-FOUR

It is impossible to recall all the special people I have dealt with as my patients in the last 10 years. Stoicism in abundance, particularly from the older generations. Bravery too from all ages, both in facing illness and sometimes death, and in dealing with disappointment and bereavement. Although I try to understand what others are going through, so I may be of some support, I don't know what it is like to lose a baby, a wife, or a parent, but to share someone's difficulties seems to help.

The day before writing these words, a brave young man whom I was lucky enough to know died at his home. In recent years his father and grandfather also died from forms of cancer, and his mother was kind enough to give me a possession of his grandfather's which depicts St Luke and a physician's prayer: 'Give skill to my hand, clear vision to my mind, kindness and sympathy to my heart. Give me singleness of purpose, strength to lift at least a part of the burden of my suffering fellow men and a true realisation of the privilege that is mine.'

And it is a privilege, to be entrusted by someone with their own or their family's health, such as their little baby about whom they may be worried sick. It is down to the GP to do their utmost for that child, and to help the parents who can, 10 minutes after arriving at the surgery, go home with their worry eased, even if at times the GP's is increased. One of my consultant colleagues asked how we cope, after he called his doctor to examine their sick child, who was pretty ill with a temperature of 40 degrees. The GP diagnosed a viral illness, which was correct, but how could he sleep thinking that the youngster could be starting with meningitis or another lethal condition, he asked.

For someone to have confidence in you, and to feel that you can make a difference to their lives, is a great honour. Sometimes, of course, you can't make a difference. Some people have incurable diseases, and some just lead miserable lives. Poverty, family troubles, and certain types of personality are difficult for a doctor to do anything about. Some poor souls just keep turning up hoping you can do something. Your heart can sink in frustration for them – and yourself. I have a box of tissues by my desk, in case my distressed patients cry. I think it makes them realise that they are not the only patients who get upset. (It also comes in handy for my horrendous colds which I catch from my patients on a regular basis.)

Perhaps just being there helps at times. Often the people whom you haven't helped are the most grateful. I get embarrassed, though touched, by the presents and cards I get, both for myself and Carole and the kids.

The emotional rewards are the greatest of all. To share in someone's happiness is exhilarating and uplifting. The relief when someone critically ill comes through. The joy when a precious baby is born, and the gratitude I feel when an honour is given, such as being made godfather to a special little girl.

Medicine is never dull. I can say I have hardly ever been bored at any time during my career. The only time I watch the clock is to wonder where the time goes. In fact, I watch the clock far too much, as if I have to run to keep up with everything I have to do. There is a great deal of unpredictability in the work. One can be lulled into a false sense of complacency, then suddenly the phone rings and an urgent visit comes through, and the day's routine evaporates. Fortunately, most of those left twiddling their thumbs in the waiting room appreciate one can be unavoidably delayed. One has to expect the unexpected and learn to live with uncertainty.

Medicine is detective work. Being given a jumbled set of symptoms and signs and trying to figure out what on earth is going on can be fascinating. Admittedly, the coughs and colds don't stretch one's abilities too greatly, though they can be important to the person presenting with them.

Medicine is worrying. One earns one's money in medicine, not because of the training, the hours, or the skill, but for the worry. The fact that you can see a patient and give them your best attention but can never be certain that you have got it right, greys the doctor's hair, furrows the brow, and generally ages us. Many doctors go home thinking, 'Could I have done anything different there? Will they be okay at home?' The buck stops with you, the GP. Although you haven't got a colleague with you on a visit to someone's home, you have got a partner in their care – your patient. If they are happy with your management then usually you are.

Medicine has many other roles. Someone's ally in times of difficulty, be it as social worker, family, or even spiritual helper. So long as you care. My retired partner and friend suggested this was the most important factor of all: to care. Seeing over 50 people in a day can be wearing, shifting your attention from one case to another every eight minutes or so. It takes stamina, and for this you have to like people, to get on with them, and to laugh *with* them and not *at* them.

Many often, in fact, have a laugh at *me*. Children, particularly, are the great levellers. Priding myself on my communication skills, or perhaps because their intelligence is similar to mine, I have been guilty of talking down to them.

Early on in my work I reviewed a six-year-old girl who had been quite poorly with a chest infection. Raising my eyebrows and with a ridiculous smile on my face I asked this thriving child, now radiating good health, 'Are you feeling better now?'

'Of course I am, you berk,' came the reply. Immaturity comes even more easily when dealing with younger children. Having left my own kindergarten at home, singing 'Postman Pat' and 'Fireman Sam' on my arrival to work in the morning, I can communicate in several different dialects of gibberish. Most youngsters appreciate my efforts to put them at their ease, though some seem to want to consult someone more sensible. I have a small blackboard at kids' level on the wall in my surgery, and a large poster on the ceiling above my examination couch with a cat dancing in the rain saying, 'Don't worry! Be happy!' This is probably appallingly superficial to someone who thinks they have cancer, but to many of all ages who lie spread-eagled on my couch I understand it at least gives them something to focus on.

I also have something to focus on. On the wall where my gaze falls in between, and occasionally during, consultations are a couple of photos of my little family, which remind me what I am doing it all for. Most patients comment on how the kids are growing, though occasionally one or two of the blokes comment how they wouldn't mind being married to Carole. Quite a few enquire how we all are, having shared our trials and tribulations along the way. In fact, it surprises me how many of my patients are kind enough to ask how I am. On occasions they have found out, as doctors make hopeless patients, and demonstrate dramatically their medical weaknesses. Part of this is because we are sometimes at work when we shouldn't be. Diarrhoea and vomiting, chest infections, bad backs … I've had and worked with the lot, as have most doctors.

When one doesn't leave the same room for three or more hours at a time you have to be resourceful. Unfortunately, I am not. Hence, for example, taking effervescent painkillers for a virus infection without a glass of water can be a problem. What happens is the tablets fizz on your tongue, then your cheeks blow out then bubbles start coming out of your nose. Then you desperately try to swallow the tablets and get uncontrollable flatulence. My patient who walked into this scenario must have thought I had rabies.

More recently a kindly man who was just three weeks after a heart attack almost relapsed on walking into my surgery to see me hunched up in agony holding my left arm, just as he had done recently. In fact, I had stretched prior to his coming in, and re-dislocated my left shoulder again. There are times when I consider having my shoulder repaired, but having retired from windsurfing and, more importantly, being a coward, I have shied away from an operation. Besides, it reminds the kids that even I am not indestructible.

Driving down our road recently they were being particularly stubborn about fixing their seatbelts as we set off. I leaned awkwardly backwards to force them to click them into place, and out popped my shoulder. I crawled out of the car, in pain, and stood hunched on the pavement. At this point a concerned man in his sixties rushed out to ask if I was okay. On hearing what the trouble was he informed me that there was a doctor who lived down the avenue. He was aghast when I told him that I *was* that doctor, but he soon recovered his composure enough to tell me about his arthritic knees.

Out and about and at the surgery I have felt flummoxed on a number of occasions when I have unexpectedly encountered someone I should have known, but unless that person's notes are directly in front of me, I have felt like a fish out of water. Hundreds of names whizz in and out of the brain, but not the name of the person in question. Having then been requested to write a prescription, wild guesses about the person's name can be made, or alternatively I clutch inanely at straws by saying something like, 'Could you just remind me how to spell your first name?'

Occasionally this works, but on the last occasion I tried it, the lady's name was Ruth. Making any further excuses is futile, as the patient then becomes worried that their doctor can't spell names with more than three letters.

On other occasions I have been informed how people's nearest and dearest are faring, when I haven't a clue who they are talking about. For some years my polite acknowledgement as someone I knew walked by in the street would be, 'Hello, how are you?' This is a very bad phrase for a local GP to make, as the person usually tells you. Symptoms and signs may be given to you even without asking, and I remember one morning walking back to the local video shop, with a rather thick head from some wine the night before, when a lady shot out of one of the side streets to inform me that her period had just started, and proceeded to tell me the amount and consistency.

I used to worry that I would be expected to behave in a certain stereotyped way within the local community, never being seen looking unfit, or drinking in a local pub, in case people felt this wasn't correct. Now it doesn't bother me, as no one seems to mind. Being a noticeable member of the populace can have its drawbacks, however, and the line has to be drawn somewhere. A year or two after arriving in the town, I collected some photos from a New Year's Eve spent with friends. As I pored over the snaps I was horrified to arrive at one which showed a penis hanging out of a pair of trousers. One contemporary of mine had taken a self-portrait after I had retired to bed and not told me! How I prayed that no one in the shop knew me.

The main venue at which I am spotted these days is our local Tesco. I often take the kids to 'help'. We end up buying all sorts of things I didn't intend to, and people rush up to help us at the checkout, in a usually futile attempt to get us out of the shop as fast as possible. Another problem GPs find, is that when one is stocking up with high cholesterol foods and alcohol, one is noticed by a particularly large number of patients that day.

I think my brain must be getting full, as I am prone to welcome patients into my surgery, and ask how I can help, only to be told that they are there at my request, if only I could remember why. Worse is when patients fool their GP by coming in in the wrong order, and the GP starts the consultation thinking they are talking to someone with a completely different medical history than they actually have. Not very confidence-inspiring. It is difficult to know instantaneously all 2,400 patients on my list, even after 10 years, but after a couple more decades perhaps I'll know everyone.

Being thorough, and I suppose in some ways still slightly obsessional, I frequently refer to my *British National Formulary* medicines guide beside me in surgery, to check doses, drug interactions, or even, 'What on earth am I going to prescribe here?' Nowadays, of course, we have to check cost too.

Our practice prescribes over one million pounds worth of drugs per year, using other people's money. It behoves us to be accountable.

Some outside medicine would no doubt say perhaps too much money goes on doctors' salaries. I don't forget that the average GP's NHS income, which is supposed to be over £40,000 per year, is a larger sum than many people get. I have argued that most earn it. Three times the national average for suicides, divorce, and alcoholism are not statistics which occur by chance. The pressure can be considerable, and though 'burn-out' is a fashionable phrase, too many GPs and doctors in other walks of life know too much about it from personal experience. In fact, we are only just getting used to the idea of looking after ourselves, so that we can look after others.

Day after day, year after year and, for some patients, decade after decade of care requires a commitment. The job satisfaction can be immense though, and towards the end of one's career to be looking after the children of women who themselves were brought into the world with one's assistance earlier in the same career, must be wonderful. General practice is a way of life, for life.

CHAPTER TWENTY-FIVE

In the summer of 1994, Carole and I pushed our luck just once more. So happy were we with Tom and Adam, and realising we were getting to the ages where pregnancies become more complicated, which in our case was a very worrying thought, we decided to have another go. Besides, perhaps this occasion would be different, and Carole would have an easier time.

No chance. At seven weeks pregnant Carole started to bleed heavily. We both knew, though neither of us would admit it to each other, that with the amount of blood she was losing, the chance of the pregnancy continuing was very small. Off we went to hospital, and one of our longest nights passed.

The next morning, to our surprise and relief, an ultrasound scan showed there was a tiny little foetus hanging on in there, along with a blood clot that was as big as he or she was. We will never know what happened. It is possible there was a second gestation sac, a very early second foetus, a twin – who didn't make it.

Serial scans followed, while our little baby got gradually bigger and the blood clot got smaller. Carole must have been truly sick of my asking how her loss was, hardly the romance of years ago, but slowly the bleeding settled and she began to look pregnant. Even more screening tests were available during this pregnancy than with Tom and Adam, which sometimes can pose more questions than answers. When asked if we wanted to know the sex of our baby, we declined. So that none of Carole's friends or colleagues would accidentally tell her, the results were locked in the hospital safe, so hardly anyone knew – except possibly a burglar who some weeks later broke in!

While my colleagues and patients know me to be someone who encourages normal childbirth where possible, we felt that after all the uncertainties neither of us could take much more, so we thought about ways to encourage Mr Wright to perform a caesarean section in this case. I wanted to draw a dotted line across Carole's lower abdomen with 'Cut Here' and a pair of scissors drawn on but she declined.

In the event, and by persuading him that this way he could also ensure we never troubled him obstetrically again, Max was born by caesarean section on 6 March 1995, the day before I became 36 years old, the best birthday present I ever had.

His older brothers thought this was great, and they were wonderful with him and desperate to hold him. They were far more at ease with him than I think I was with my younger brothers when they were tiny. History had repeated itself. Three more Barker boys, with almost exactly the same age gap between them as myself and my brothers.

Another spring baby. Warm nights, early dawns, blossoming trees, and colourful flowers, seen through bleary bloodshot but happy eyes. Perhaps because I knew, barring the small failure rate I always counsel people about, that Max would be our last child, I minded even less getting up in the night – or perhaps I was just conditioned to it by then!

Maybe my mental age is regressing even further. After Max was born I arranged for a ten-foot wooden blue stork to be erected overlooking our front garden wall, with Max's date of arrival and weight on. Carole says that on arriving home she almost burst her stitches with embarrassment.

Since then friends have told me that, if they were given the names of a hundred people and asked which one would plant a ridiculously large bird in their garden, it would undoubtedly be me. With any luck, I'll grow up with my children so that I might not be such an embarrassment to them when they are older. As an antidote to the seriousness of work, I love coming home and letting off steam with the kids, and at times I think Carole feels she has four sons.

I certainly do not intend to miss our kids growing up, so I spend as much time as possible with them when I am off. Occasionally, I am reminded of how I would like to be there for them more often. Before Max arrived, Tom came home with a drawing on a t-shirt of a mummy and two boys.

'Where am I?' I demanded.

'At work,' he replied.

I've learned a lot from our boys, and this knowledge has probably helped me at work. I know what it is like to be exhausted with crying babies, to worry they have some desperate illness when logic suggests it's a mild cold. I used to frown and knowledgeably decline a request from a tired mum for something to help a toddler sleep, just for a night or two. Now, living in the real world, I am more flexible. Having scoured the local paper to find out which emergency chemist is open to buy a dummy for Tom in his infancy, and then to find he didn't want it, I know what frustration is. Transferring babes from breast to bottle, with every shaped teat available, can be harrowing too. If some of these are supposed to be nipple-shaped, then there are some odd-shaped nipples around. Trying to remain calm together when your baby is screaming can be difficult.

'Leave him, he'll be okay.'

'I can't, he's unhappy.'

'He's fed, changed and fine.'

'I still can't leave him,' Carole would say, lactating everywhere.

Patients seem to value my opinion as a dad at least as much as my opinion as a doctor. I can say, 'Yes, I would have my kids vaccinated,' because I have. Only today, however, during the child health surveillance clinic my limitations were yet again exposed. A worried mum wanted to discuss the measles/mumps/rubella vaccination. As she asked me if I'd had my baby vaccinated, the realisation dawned that at two o'clock that afternoon Max was supposed to have his vaccination, and I had forgotten. Send in the social workers, alert the health visitors. I admitted my error and took home the vaccine to give myself.

However, I didn't give it straight away, because Carole is on her own with the kids tonight. Right now, as I write the first draft of my book, it is 2.52am and I am working for the medical co-operative between midnight and seven in the morning. We have had five calls so far: colic, diarrhoea and vomiting, abdominal pain, a viral illness, and one other.

Out of the blue we got a call to a woman who'd had a cardiac arrest. My navigator got us there in eight minutes, the paramedics had arrived before us and intubated her and got a venous line in. With further cardiopulmonary resuscitation we got her round, and she was admitted to intensive care. I have since learned that she died.

Two more calls as day dawned, then home to bed on this occasion, as what time I haven't spent seeing patients I have been writing this. A twelve-hour day, followed by four hours of 'rest' putting the kids to bed, then seven hours' night work, leaves me tired. I must be getting old. On the occasions

I have tried to stay up the whole of the following day, I usually embarrass Carole by falling asleep wherever we are the next evening. This leaves her to make excuses that I am not bored with whoever's company we are in, nor have I been drinking excessively.

One morning recently, after working during the night, I felt too high to go to bed, so I sat assessing the health of our financial situation, with a view to moving house. Tom was first to get up and stumbled sleepily into the room.

'What are you doing, Dad?' said Tom.

'Working out if we have enough money to buy a house Mummy and Daddy have seen.'

'Will this help?' he said, giving me a one pound coin the tooth fairy had left him during the night.

'Thanks, Tom, but we'll need an awful lot more than that.'

'Well, I could take all my teeth out!'

When I am somewhat worn down by life's serious situations, I get great strength from the honesty and naivety of our children, occasionally hankering after a time when I was like that myself.

With one look or one word, kids can take you up to a glorious high, then crash you back down again. On holiday recently, I was doing my best to manage the carnage that was teatime with Tom and Adam, while Carole nursed Max who had a nasty ear infection. A couple of elderly ladies came up to our table and said to me, 'We've been watching you, and we think you make a wonderful father.' For a microsecond I beamed with pride, only for Adam to shout 'What!?', as if he couldn't possibly imagine somebody saying that to his dad. I'd like to think he was, in fact, enquiring what the elderly ladies had said, but probably not.

Earlier that day I had taken a lovely family photograph, with the camera on self-timer, of the five of us sat together. Unfortunately, just as the shutter opened, Max vomited profusely, and the photo in fact consists of the four of us turning our heads to our poorly little one.

I have built up quite a collection of photographs over the years, and have bored countless people, both taking photographs, and showing them.

Adam again, looking through photos of Carole and me: 'Where am I in the picture?'

'You hadn't been born yet.'

'I was in Mummy's tummy?'

'Not even in Mummy's tummy.'

'You mean,' he said with a quizzical look, 'I was nowhere?'

Eight years ago they were nowhere but, as we explained to the kids, because Mummy and Daddy met and love each other so much, they were made. Now they are everywhere. If I died tomorrow I would be thoroughly annoyed, but I would feel at least I've left a part of me behind in three little Barkers.

I don't know how long I'll be around. If statistics are anything to go by, which they aren't, I've had half of my life. I certainly feel good for many miles yet. I have given up water sports, and intend to look after myself. I have slimmed down to 12 stone, from 13.5 in recent years. I don't smoke, and I drink in moderation (usually). I've had the occasional heart rhythm disturbance, an SVT, or even atrial fibrillation, but then many people do – only they are not so introspective as to have an ECG tracing done.

In fact, I try to analyse matters less than I used to, and concentrate more on getting on with life and enjoying it. My patients tell me that the older one becomes, the quicker time passes. I am already finding this, as the time taken for Tom and Adam to progress through each year at school seems far less than it was when I was at their stage in life. Already they are past the earliest years that I can recall of my schooling, and their experiences now will be forming their characters and ways of approaching life.

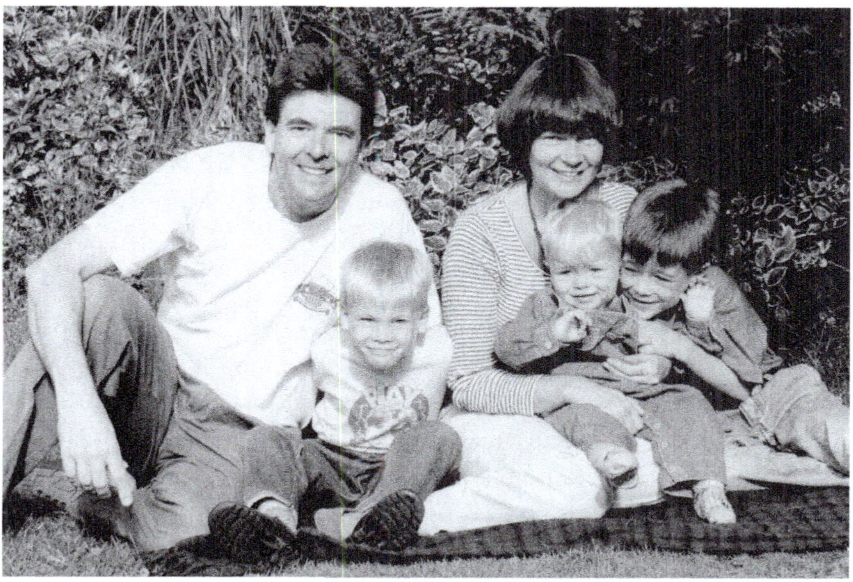

Me, Adam, Carole, Max and Tom, 1996

They are fortunate enough to attend an excellent local county primary school where the teachers' dedication is inspiring. We live one and a half miles away, and when we applied for Tom to be admitted the school was oversubscribed, for the first time ever, by one. Hence, following in his father's footsteps, Tom was unsuccessful in the initial application. Carole and I drew up a huge list of reasons why Tom should be admitted, but before the appeal a place became available anyway. We were informed of this by a letter from the local education authority, stating that, 'Our daughter Victoria could now attend.' Shades of Olive here. Although we were keen, we weren't going to put him in a dress and pretend he was female, so I enquired and fortunately there had been a mix up of names, and Tom was after all allowed in.

Since then we have proudly witnessed his and Adam's school progress. We are told at parents' evenings of these mild-mannered, polite little angels who at times do not quite resemble the strong-willed hyperactive whirlwinds we know and love at home. Even little Max has his own phrases now. Less than a week after having a new bathroom carpet put down, I turned my shaver off to hear below me Max saying 'Oh Max, oh Max,' in exactly the way Carole and I chastise him. He was purposefully emptying a tube of blue gel Mickey Mouse toothpaste in a little circle on to our recent purchase.

Where they get their energy from I don't know. I am barely through the front door in the evenings before being greeted with, 'Daddy, can we play football?' Then Max comes bounding up, face beaming, equally keen to join in. Work is quickly forgotten, and all four of us hurtle around inside or out, depending on the weather and how good they've been. If Carole is not at work, then she has almost a minute's respite, before getting stuck into all the things she has tried to do so far that day, but has been physically prevented.

We have made some very good friends through our kids, though as we chat at various events and parties requiring our chauffeuring services, we already see the pace of our offspring's social lives outstripping our own.

Underfunding of state schools has caused considerable difficulty nationwide, and we have been able to experience this first-hand. Many of us wrote to our MP and the local education authority about the situation which was soon to cause some of the school's teachers to be made redundant. The politicians blamed the local education authority and vice versa, and we got nowhere. So Alison, another parent, and I went to the LEA to ask directly what was going on, and what support the teachers were getting. The debate that ensued involving them, the governors, teachers, MP, and parents became increasingly heated.

A group of parents, of which Carole and I were part, became referred to by some as 'rebels and troublemakers'. This was deeply hurtful as we were only trying to do the best for our children and their teachers. Our consciences would not let us sit and do nothing. In fact, in retrospect, I probably said less than I could have done, yet again trying to be on everyone's side. In the end, partly due to our efforts I would like to think, fewer teachers had to leave than was originally anticipated.

As yet, the kids are not embarrassed to be seen with us, and we all join in the fundraising activities, such as treasure hunts and summer fairs, where Carole and I this year sold 250 synthetic-looking (and tasting) hot dogs, to unsuspecting but very charitable punters.

I was recently touched to be asked to come in and talk to Adam's class about what it was like to be a doctor, in a series of talks by 'people who help'. Adam, fortunately, did not seem too troubled by this, but I am sure I was not anywhere near as fascinating as the dad who was a policeman, with accompanying police car and dog. Somehow, a stethoscope is not quite so interesting.

CHAPTER TWENTY-SIX

In my medical career so far, I feel like lightning has struck twice. I was asked to see a lady one afternoon who was unwell, and so I visited, and performed a thorough medical history and examination. In accordance with advice to get back in touch if needed, she phoned the next morning, when she had suddenly become a lot worse. Revisiting immediately, I confirmed this situation, and having called the paramedics, gave appropriate treatment and rushed her into hospital. I thought we had saved her life, but tragically she died days later.

I tried to support her family to my utmost ability, and I felt we had all become close through this grief. In fact, as sometimes happens, I was asked to the funeral.

Unfortunately, some months later, the lady's husband started legal proceedings against me. A letter arrived on my desk, alleging I had been negligent in not admitting her the first time, detailing procedures up to trial. This weighed further on my already heavy heart.

Having never previously received a complaint, I contacted my medico-legal advisers who supported me from there. What I find particularly upsetting is that once legal proceedings are commenced, barriers go up, so that the actual people involved find it more difficult to communicate. We tried, but from the tone of the first letter I received we knew it wasn't going to be easy and, after another three months, the lady's husband said he was going to register with another doctor. From then on I heard nothing, though I thought often about their loss and the pending case.

A whole year later, I received through my letterbox one of the local papers carrying details of the case. Reading with stunned and racing mind,

I tried to digest what it said. The medical expert had decided that if my lady had been admitted earlier, she would have had a better chance of survival, but also that her doctor (me) should be cleared of any blame, as events could not have been foreseen. All sorts of emotions flooded in and out of me. Most of all, though, I felt like crying for the lady herself, and for all of us, that it had come to this. I was not even party to the expert's judgement, as he was 'their' witness.

Again I phoned my medico-legal adviser, partly in case the same paper asked for my comments. I presumed that at this stage I would be able to express my continued sorrow for the family's loss, but would be unable to comment further. I was advised that if I could bear it, I should not even express sorrow, in case the plaintiff's solicitors made something of it. I am sure that this was sound medico-legal advice, but it seems a shame that this is the system which at present prevails.

A detailed review of the medico-legal system has recently been published in the Wolff Report, which will hopefully lead to more satisfactory and humane arrangements. At present, people who have a grievance against their own or their family's medical practitioner have to go through months, if not years, of stressful reliving of the events, while the doctors or nurses do the same, each party distanced further and further by legal jargon, and advice not to communicate except via a solicitor's letter.

I sincerely hope, as I said in the last phone call between me and her husband some time ago now, that he and their children can find happiness in their futures, remembering a remarkable wife and mother.

CHAPTER TWENTY-SEVEN

Where is medicine, and in particular general practice going? What further changes will I see in the coming years? Politically, there are moves afoot to expand the role of general practice further, so that doctors can develop their special interests. This could be a good thing, but not many in the profession can see where the time and money to enable this to be possible is going to come from.

As it is, fewer and fewer young doctors see general practice as an attractive option, and recruitment is difficult in many areas. Compared with the sixty applicants for five places to the Preston GP Training Scheme for 1983, there were three applicants this year. None of them turned up for interview, and when the posts were re-advertised no one applied! Most GPs know of one or more of their colleagues who has had to have some time off due to work-related anxiety or depression, or just plain overwork.

Doctors are being seen as increasingly necessary resources for people to rely on, to the point of absurdity at times. We are asked by insurance companies to virtually guarantee that patients will not become ill on holiday, or collapse at their health club. Most people are happy to take responsibility for their own health, but some organisations are not. Last week, one of my partners was asked for a doctor's note to say that his patient had to have a trolley for his golf clubs in winter, for medical reasons. Soon people will need a doctor's permission to pass wind.

Increasingly, we are asked to provide medical evidence regarding mishaps such as tripping over kerb stones. While it is reasonable to want compensation for negligence, surely matters are proceeding too far when a sprain from a slightly uneven pavement results in payments from the local council, who then have to cut back yet further on services such as home helps or sheltered housing for the elderly.

The field of medicine is as exciting as ever, with new developments marching on apace. Although in the profession myself, I sometimes feel like the O-level pupil I was over 20 years ago, fascinated by episodes of the science documentary programme *Horizon*. Attending lectures on how electronic engineering techniques could help overcome some neurological failure or sensory deprivation is fascinating, as is learning how microsurgery can aid the penetration of an ovum by a sperm, or how genetic engineering is leading to gene therapy for conditions such as cystic fibrosis.

I am privileged to be able to witness such progress, but I try not to forget that this is not the world most people live in. Worldwide, every day there are between 30,000 and 40,000 child deaths from diseases related to malnutrition. Hundreds of millions of the world's population live in dreadful poverty. Health for all has been described as a distant dream. Perhaps in our children's, or our children's children's generations this goal may be a little more tangible.

What will my children think when their time to choose careers arrives? I hope we will encourage them wisely, to do whatever they choose. I wouldn't advise them to follow a career in medicine, but then I don't think I would actively discourage them either, though it is interesting that none of my partners' children, and very few practising GPs' children, it seems, follow in their parents' footsteps. Perhaps this is because they see the more serious side of a GP's life – the hours and the worry.

The lighter side often isn't seen, and mostly can't be discussed in detail for confidentiality reasons, or perhaps because most medical people see their experiences from a different angle than others might.

Many of the strange tales we encounter lose a lot in the telling. It is difficult to describe how bizarre one can feel trying to carry out a home consultation with the patient's parrot on your shoulder squawking throughout. Or to hide one's resignation on enquiring of a patient, 'How is your hearing?' and they reply loudly, 'What?!' Or being told, as one of my pals was when visiting a patient and remarking how beautiful the views were, 'I've been blind for twenty years.'

Equally embarrassing situations occur regularly. Another of my contemporaries was recently consulted by a patient with acne. Thinking she had just the thing for this, she gave him a free sample of a product given to her by a pharmaceutical representative. Unfortunately the box did not contain the acne treatment as she thought, but a magnifying glass! No wonder his mum phoned up confused as to what they were to do with it.

Extraordinary situations sometimes occur with those suffering from delusions or psychotic states. I have seen someone literally tear wallpaper off the walls in a manic state. People in these conditions can spend phenomenal amounts of money unintentionally, or reorganise their whole house, garden, family and pets without knowing what they are doing. Trying to persuade sufferers that they need help can be exceedingly difficult.

Many GPs have transported such patients to hospital personally, as we have been the only ones they would trust when so disturbed. Some people find amusement in such incidents – including, at times, the sufferers themselves when better – but it is an acutely upsetting experience for the patient and their family at the time, and they need all the support they can get.

Bizarre tales are told, which could be apocryphal, but I doubt it, such as when a farmer asked his passing GP to help put a dying sheep out of its misery. Perhaps unwisely, the GP administered a large dose of morphine, upon which the sheep became high, and acquired a new lease of life! Perhaps I am gullible, but I am interested to hear the tales of others. Some years ago my brother Alec succeeded in getting another one over on me by saying, 'Do you realise that the word "gullible" isn't in the English dictionary?'

I replied, 'Isn't it?'

Fortunately, I am less easily persuaded at work, and concerning patients with drug- and alcohol-related problems, I am less easily fooled than I was 10 years ago. These are particularly testing areas of practice, though most do not mean to be malicious, even if some can be deceitful at times.

Intoxicated patients can present problems in surgery, partly because when they leave the consulting room, the next patient doesn't seem sure whether or not it is their GP who is emanating the overpowering fumes. In fact, by the end of a hot week my room has a combination of interesting odours, particularly feet, that are probably dangerously inflammable!

Drug-related problems are a difficult area for the primary health care team, and at times medical and nursing professionals are seen as easy targets for drugs. Most of the medications in our bags, however, would not induce enjoyable states of mind at all. At best they would be sedative, and at worst potentially dangerous when used inappropriately.

Thanks to our local community we have not had to put fortress-like armaments around our surgery, though it is multiple-locked and alarmed and linked to the nearby police headquarters. (This has proved somewhat irksome recently, as on three occasions I have had to attend after the alarm has been set off by spiders.) I would like to think that folk are aware that we are only trying to give a service to local people, and that breaking into a surgery or assaulting the local GP or nurse is not going to achieve much. Sadly, this does happen in some, particularly inner city, areas. In fact, I was also recently left in no doubt about the degree of respect that the medical profession is held in by some. A car was being broken into just outside the confines of our car park by a youth who was clearly rattled as I leapt over the wall shouting at him. He retorted, 'F*** off, knobhead,' obviously awestruck by my presence.

Only once, as far as I am aware, has one of my practice partners been near to being assaulted, and that was when one of my partners was mistaken for another!

On one occasion, I was concerned when someone told me that, if he was not satisfied by an enquiry, he was 'ex army.' Fortunately, he *was* satisfied, though I am under no illusion about the strength of feeling people have about the medical care they and their loved ones receive. Recently, a GP in Scotland was murdered by a relative of a patient who had died some years before, in spite of not being to blame for that death. The nature of the job is such that we can all expect to face verbal, if not physical threats at some time in our working lives.

CHAPTER TWENTY-EIGHT

Although fewer doctors have entered general practice in recent years, some hospital specialities are proving increasingly popular, and now many of my medical school contemporaries are consultants in their own fields. At our 10-year reunion in 1992, those of us in general practice were more established and possibly slightly more affluent. At our 20year reunion the reverse will be true. I will have to hire an expensive car in which to arrive, to compete with some of my orthopaedic or general surgical contemporaries.

The friends I see from university and early hospital days are mostly GPs themselves. Every few Fridays a handful of us meet up in Manchester to have a drink and moan about work. Some regions have 'young practitioners groups', but this has two disadvantages. One is that no one can decide when a member stops being 'young', and the other is that discussing problems with people one doesn't know too well can be difficult. With good friends of many years I feel totally comfortable and relaxed, and enjoy my fix of laughter therapy. With friends like Ewan and Danny and Brian, whose senses of humour are even more bizarre than my own, my sides literally ache after an hour or two. I am only too well aware that I don't share their sparkle, but perhaps act as a catalyst for getting people together every now and then.

Once a year, Danny and Dermot and Richard and I go golfing to play for the Ulrika Jonsson trophy. Before our first trip to Scotland we avidly watched the weather forecasts on TV. At that time this attractive blonde Scandinavian was presenting the bulletins, and we naturally decided that the prize should be some time in Ms Jonsson's company.

The winner that year wrote to her, and to her credit she wrote back enclosing a signed photograph. Hence at the end of each weekend we have a ceremony where that year's winner is presented with the framed photograph. The other hotel residents look enquiringly on, witnessing this rather pathetic ritual. The one year I won, she lasted all of 10 seconds on the mantelpiece, before Tom came upstairs saying, 'Mummy says put this in your bottom drawer.'

Now Tom is seven. At his recent birthday party he had ten guests. Four pretty, polite, demure well-behaved girls, and six lads who, incited partly by him, went absolutely wild! Food fights and general mayhem for two hours.

I try to do my best for our kids and their friends, though already I am beginning to see that one's intentions and words can be somewhat misinterpreted. Recently, Tom and Adam, along with Max, had a school photograph taken. What remained of Tom's two front teeth had come out some months ago, and he has a large expectant gap where his adult teeth have yet to come through. I suggested that he would still look handsome if he gave a big smile with his mouth closed. I remember not being fond of photos taken of myself at a similar stage. On the way to school for the photograph Tom announced to Carole that Daddy thought his mouth looked horrible, which is not quite how I had intended it to be interpreted.

On another occasion, one of Tom's bright mischievous friends came round to play, and mysteriously one of our door keys went missing. After making enquiries of Tom and his friend I was none the wiser, but suggested to Carole that I would like to be around next time to keep an eye on things. On arriving at school the next day Tom announced to his friend that he was not allowed to come and play unless Dad was around 'because he says you steal things!' Fortunately, I am still on good terms with him and his parents.

With three sons I seem to be perpetually living the first five minutes of the popular television programme *Casualty*. At the beginning of each episode, boisterous games are taking place in relative innocence, yet the viewer knows some disaster is about to ensue.

Actually, so far, we have been very lucky. The only upsetting injury was on our first night abroad after becoming parents, where Tom, being a Barker boy and therefore developmentally slow, had only just learned to walk at 15 months. He missed a step, while yours truly was supposed to be looking after him, and smashed both his front upper teeth.

We still go abroad on holiday, when time and finances allow, and from the warm comfort of my armchair, I enjoy looking back on the way some of the expeditions I, and previously my father, have taken our respective families on. It is easy to forget what it is like to feel cold, wet, lost and with blistered feet.

At the age of about twelve, my two young brothers and I set off with Dad to walk the twenty plus miles that are the Yorkshire Three Peaks, in school shoes and with a packet of biscuits. Halfway up Whernside we got lost, gave up, and walked even further than we were meant to, toiling our way back to our campsite. I ran on ahead to prepare camp for our return, but almost unintentionally copied Captain Oates, as the other three were picked up shortly after by a Jeep driver who took pity on them.

Even after meeting Carole I hadn't learned my lesson. With a group of friends we set off on a bright spring day to walk up Mount Snowdon. How we laughed at the posers coming down the mountain with helmets and ice axes, when any fool knows a train goes up that hill, so it couldn't possibly be a serious climb. Two hours later I had that familiar lost feeling (if that isn't a contradiction in terms). As the cloud came down, we encountered snow, and discovered that ropes were in fact needed on the steeper slopes. I would have chastised Carole for wearing flimsy 'nature trekker' shoes, if I hadn't been wearing a jacket which was about as waterproof as one of those cheesecloth shirts I used to wear in the 1970s.

Slowly but surely, as with so many things, Carole has steered me in another direction. In our early holidays together I still used to get blistered feet, only this time due to forgetting to put sun cream on them. We used to laze around frying slowly, cooling off with chilled white wine or sangria. Unfortunately, we used to regularly overdo the cooling off on the last night of our holiday.

In France, Carole left the showerhead dripping over the outside of the bath all night, so the next morning as I stumbled into the bathroom of our gîte, head pounding, my feet squelched even more loudly than my stomach. The water on the floor seeped down to the garage below, as Ewan and I went to inform the owner, Madame Quenon, '*Nous avons une petite problème. Votre maison est dans l'eau.*'

In Spain we kept ourselves to ourselves for two weeks, then on the last night had a party, at which I finally admitted my occupation. This is normally a closely guarded secret on holiday, so as to avoid being quizzed about all sorts of conditions – and also in case I behave less than maturely. On that holiday, the latter involved spontaneously stripping down to my underwear at two o'clock in the morning and diving into the swimming pool to cool off and sober up. Necks have been broken by others less fortunate doing exactly that.

We then had to drive for two days through arid southern Spain, worsening our dehydration and cerebral function. Nowhere was this more obvious than on a Friday afternoon rush-hour in Malaga, while we searched in vain for some of the hotels Carole was sure were there when she was last in that city. Unfortunately she was thinking of Magaluf, in Majorca, which explains why we circled the docks for hours on end finding not a single resting place.

Children bring a whole new series of perils to be encountered on holiday. One of the first, and definitely the most embarrassing, was the baby-listening service. On our first hotel holiday as parents, this allowed us to leave Tom sleeping peacefully while we enjoyed a relatively civilised dinner together. The microphone above our bed relayed any noise to the hotel reception. On the one night we weren't too exhausted to fall into a deep sleep immediately after getting into bed, I forgot to switch it off. The next morning we realised this, and took particular care to avoid any inquisitive or knowing glances, and denied vehemently that we were anything to do with 'the couple from Room 42'.

Shortly after that we spent a few days at one of the Center Parcs locations. While I am sure these are wonderful for families with older children, to take a boy of two and one of barely six months, in November, was not one of our best ideas. The indoor tropical swimming pool acted as a culture medium for all sorts of interesting bacteria that would soon find their way into our children's upper respiratory tracts. Having then endured profusely snotty, pyrexial and grumpy children on this trip, Carole virtually comes up in an allergic reaction to the very mention of the place.

On holiday these days with three children, we feel like United Nations negotiators trying to please everyone all of the time. Carole is very patient, as her four boys trip off to theme parks and play areas, consuming vast amounts of junk food as we go. One needs the wisdom of Solomon to decide who gets what, how, where and when. I have great plans for Florida, Seattle, and Australia in the coming years – but are *they* ready for *us*?

While I enjoy observing worried-looking passengers getting on various planes, casting sickening looks in our direction as they realise they are seated near the 'family from hell', two or three hours with our tribe may be manageable, but more may not be so easy!

CHAPTER TWENTY-NINE

Holidays may be somewhat limited in the coming year, as we are currently involved in house-moving, having partially wrecked the house we now live in. According to many, moving home is the third most stressful life event, after the death of a first-degree relative, then divorce. Writing this book has taken up a relatively minuscule amount of time and money compared to our attempt to up sticks two miles, yet at times has seemed to achieve considerably more!

A year ago, Carole and I saw a house we liked the look of, and hence put our own up for sale. What a doddle, we thought, as an offer came in after a week, though this was for considerably less than we were asking. Perhaps this was because within days of our sign going up, a van arrived at a house just down the road with 'Subsidence Services' written on the side! We turned down this offer, and now are in a position over a year later to have to accept the second offer we received, which is for less, having lost the house we originally wanted.

Not only that, but within three weeks of planning to move to the house we eventually found, although our offer had been accepted down to the Wendy house, one of the vendors had second thoughts about selling. Having spent the last five months playing the roles of assistant solicitor, estate agent, and marriage guidance counsellor, we were thousands of pounds worse off, and yet had moved almost absolutely nowhere.

It was just as well I am used to breaking bad news to people, as all my skills were called on to inform our purchasers, who were fairly understanding, but who eventually gave us an ultimatum to move or lose our sale. We were therefore committed to leaving our dear home of nine years, even though we did not have a firm date on which we could move into our new home.

We had to move, as I don't think our previous abode could take much more of my DIY skills. As winter drew in, it was difficult to see at night from the back door, as we no longer had an outside light there. Some time ago I realised the bulb needed replacing. On removing the lantern-effect glass, the metalwork disintegrated. On attempting to repair it, the bracket came away from the wall. On attempting to repair that, a brick came out of the wall – and Carole suggested I should stop there, in case the wall or even the whole house would then need replacing.

We probably got more light than most, during the day anyway, as there could be a small hole in the ozone layer above that house. When defrosting our fridge, I became aware that a small iceberg had seemingly chemically bonded to the inside of the icebox. Carole saw me trying to dislodge this with a carving knife, and correctly (again!) chastised me and suggested I used a more sensible implement. This I did, but got nowhere, so when she had gone to bed I found an even sharper carving knife to use. As Carole was dozing off, she was awoken by a loud bang, and an expletive from me, whose head disappeared in a cloud of CFCs.

Now I am more patient with such matters, though still have the occasional accident, for example trimming through the flex of our neighbour's electric hedge trimmer, and then inspecting it too closely before unplugging it from the mains.

STOP PRESS: Late November 1996.

We've moved at last!

With just days to go, various contracts were exchanged on both properties. In a whirlwind we packed up all our belongings, and transported them to what the estate agent described as a spacious six-bedroomed converted mill. In fact, since then, we have more frequently heard it described as 'the old weaving shed'! Several older local folk apparently lost their hearing working with all the machinery within, for years on end.

It has been snowing, Max has been sleepless, recovering from chicken pox and, worst of all, Carole has broken her ankle packing, but we've done it!

Helped by family and friends, we are settled in what should be our new home for the next 30 years. Even my patients have helped. A chap gave me some flowers for Carole (which caused his wife some concern when Carole wrote to thank him), and a lady has lent her a brass bell to ring when she needs anything!

And now Carole finally has space to hide away in her own little bathroom. Although we don't like to think of ourselves as 'en suite people', she has enough room to declare one small male-free zone, away from the sweaty socks, underpants, and splashes round the toilet seat!

CHAPTER THIRTY

It is difficult to know where to end this book, as events keep happening all around us. In many ways I suppose this is good, as I would hate to think that at any time in one's life something is not evolving and progressing. In fact, I have become aware towards the end of my writing, that in some ways it resembles a diary, as we move through 1996.

It may become apparent to the reader that the initially clearer boundaries between medicine and my life outside that field have become more blurred as time goes by. This could be because the direction and definition of this book and its various parts have got lost. I would like to think, however, that it is because the ways of life and medicine merge, each increasingly influencing the other.

There are happy events, such as the blooming in her second pregnancy of a lady who tragically had a stillborn babe a year ago.

There are sad events, such as the untimely death this weekend of a good man, both a patient and a neighbour of mine, who only three weeks ago rushed some flowers to Carole from his shop, following my phone call from the golfing weekend.

There are upsetting events, such as a baby who has become poorly, the reasons for which are unclear, and whose parents along with the rest of us look for answers that aren't there.

There are embarrassing events, such as my delivery of a harvest festival gift for some of the older ladies and gentleman who live around the kids' school. Most of these had involved baskets of fruit or vegetables, but at my last call, the basket was laden with pots of jam, peanut butter, and a tin of treacle sponge pudding.

'It's Dr Barker, isn't it?' enquired the recipient.

'Yes, where do I know you from?' I enquired.

'Your diabetic clinic!'

There are humorous events, on a lighter note. One of my pals was reminded recently of the need to make himself understood, and consult in plain English. When a man attended complaining of urinary symptoms, his GP asked (along with other questions) if he'd had casual sex recently. The patient replied that he had.

'How many times, in the last month or so?' asked the doctor.

'About eight or nine times,' came the reply.

'With how many different women?' came the doctor's somewhat startled response.

'Oh, always with the wife, of course!'

In no way am I trying to make light of the serious aspects of my work but, as described above, the variety of challenges presented and the care one needs to give, is the very essence of general medical practice.

In life outside medicine, the variety is endless. Two weeks ago, Carole and I travelled to Manchester to be interviewed as prospective contestants on the television programme *Can't Cook Won't Cook*. We have just heard that we have been successful, and will soon travel to Birmingham to record. (It would have been this week, had it not been for Carole's ankle.)

Some of my patients are hoping to catch the show on the waiting room TV, before consulting me in surgery. I only hope they have more faith in my medical skills than they will in my cooking abilities.

On reading this work through, I am aware that it has happy bits, sad bits, and many other bits, including rude bits – but that's life. I sincerely hope I have not caused anyone offence, and that none of it is taken out of context. I certainly hope I have never trivialised anyone's problems or predicament, as that was never my intent.

A lot has happened to me in 10 years of general practice. I have had a nervous breakdown, seen the partnership split, and been accused once of negligence. That one complaint in 14 years was not something I would like to go through again, though most of us will. In fact, when I started general practice the average GP faced a formal complaint once every ten years, and now I understand it is once every three years. However, I feel the positive aspects outweigh the negative ones, and even from those upsetting experiences, one can learn. Whether it is a worthwhile career is for the reader to decide. I would like to think it is.

I have been only too ready to discuss my weaknesses and limitations in this book. To be fair to myself, I should point out that nearly all of my patients and, to my knowledge, all of my colleagues are happy with what I do. At the risk of sounding conceited, I honestly believe that there will not be many doctors who practise a higher standard of medicine than I do. Although I have had patients for whom I wish things could have been different, every doctor has had similar experiences. In the last week alone, I have had two people consult, each in a distraught frame of mind, but both said they knew they could come to me because I would know what to do. Although a considerable responsibility, it is good to feel that people have faith in you.

Having said that, I don't think I am going to become famous in medicine. I don't seem to have the time or enthusiasm for a high-flying research project. 'Why the ears get bigger when men get older' or 'Why is belly-button fluff always purple' are not the kind of subjects one is asked to exotic destinations to lecture about.

Carole will no doubt witness and be part of even further strides in neonatal medicine and nursing. How she manages to organise our thriving little family, and work as a sister in the special care baby unit, I don't know. At times she must feel a long way away from the carefree girl in her twenties who left me a note with little drawings on, but as she sits in our dining room writing up projects on matters such as foetal and neonatal pain, I love and admire her even more now than I did then.

I look forward to further developments of the primary-care led NHS, though I do have some reservations about certain aspects of the way this is being achieved. On a more personal level, I look forward to building closer bonds with my colleagues and my patients, many of whom I now feel are friends too.

In less than a decade, some of my partners will be at an age where they might wish to retire, which would be a loss for their patients, and us 'junior' partners. This concerns me, as we have such a good thing going now, and I wonder how the practice will manage in years to come. If recruitment for replacement partners does not improve, the future is uncertain.

Outside medicine, it looks like I'll never get to be a rock star. I wasn't actually the oldest person at the recent Oasis concerts, but I was a very long way away from being the youngest. Astronauts just don't seem to be in demand nowadays. These dreams I will just have to live out through my children. Soon they'll be old enough for me to take to the Kennedy Space Centre and people might believe we are actually going for the kids.

Who knows what Tom, Adam, and Max will experience in the years and decades to come. So much has changed in my relatively short time. The 1960s I can't remember much about, but nor can many who were 'there', I understand. The 1970s were excessive and loud. The 1980s were greedy and selfish for some. The 1990s are supposed to be caring and sharing. The 2000s are completely unknown, and that is what makes the future exciting.

If I could change one thing about my life so far it would be to worry less. In fact, I would change little else. My father says that family history has taught him that we are each here for a little while, and within three or four generations no one will remember who we are, or have any idea about us, so we may as well enjoy it while we can.

One can still care, without worrying as much. I manage to wind down rather more easily nowadays, though I don't suppose one can ever completely switch off. Shortly before last Christmas, when off duty at three in the morning, I was phoned by our emergency service who had been requested to contact me by the police. A boy who I had seen a week previously had suddenly died, and they wondered if I had any information. Although this sadly premature death had nothing to do with what I had seen him with, one doesn't go back to sleep easily thinking about events like that.

I try to balance my life outside work and my life within it as best I can. There are times when I don't always get it right. Carole and the boys have cause to feel sometimes that I am too involved with my work, and yet there are no doubt patients who feel I am less accessible than I should be. On one occasion I remember one of my patients thinking I had deliberately left surgery early so that he had to see somebody else, but when I explained I was rushing to see my wife on the coronary care unit, he understood. In most cases we can all accommodate each other.

I try to keep my flock – multitude, bevy, or whatever the collective name for a group of patients is – healthy and happy. I try to do the same for my family, and myself. Although I no longer run marathons, or any further than I have to, I do still try to pretend I am fit. On our most recent holiday abroad I managed to swim the length of the 33-metre swimming pool underwater (deliberately), though must have looked pretty desperate afterwards as a concerned holidaymaker came up to ask me if I needed assistance.

As for the future, whether I will ever write a 'Part Two' to follow this book, I don't know. Probably all the copies of this work will gather dust and disintegrate, and I'll have gone to all this trouble for nothing! I hope perhaps someone might leaf through this for interest in years to come. I am often reminded about how transient life is when visiting my elderly patients and seeing a fading photograph on a mantelpiece of people who bear little or no resemblance to the shrinking, wrinkling, dying person they now are.

Besides, ambitions other than my amateur foray into the world of literature are more important now:

- to be there for our children, and others in our families, when they need me, as my parents were and are for me;

- to be there for my patients when they need me, and for my colleagues and friends, as they were for me;

- to be there for Carole, as she has always been there for me.

When I was ill all those years ago, I spent some time dwelling on what life was about. What is it for, and what does it mean? I think, sentimental though it may sound, it is to help others, and be happy. In Life and in Medicine, one can try to do both.

Printed in Great Britain
by Amazon

20159461R00098